57 Steps to Paradise

Finding Love in Midlife and Beyond

Patricia Lorenz

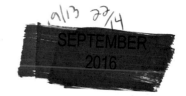

For information, contact
MSI Press
1760-F Airline Highway, #203
Hollister, CA 95023

Cover designed: Carrissa Lorenz

Cover Photo © Sergey Nivens/ShutterStock.com

Library of Congress Control Number: 2016901839

ISBN: 978-1-942891-18-5

Many of the names of the people mentioned in this book have been changed to protect their identity.

Contents

Introduction

You may be wondering why a woman on Social Security and Medicare even entertained the idea of writing a book about men. I may be middle-aged or even stumbling toward old, but I'm not dead. I like men. Men have been walking, sliding, galloping, and slithering in and out of my life for over 50 years.

We women of the biggest generation in America, the Baby Boomers, are in the majority. We outlive men. I have already outlived my second husband who left me for an older woman, married her the day of our divorce, and then died two years later in 1989.

I have no idea if I'll outlive my first husband. He's seven years older than I am, and in the years since 1975 when I left him and moved out of state after seven tortuous years together, he never remarried. If he had, perhaps he'd look younger and have a healthier lifestyle. In the years since we divorced, he's had some tough medical problems so who knows which one of us will check out first.

I also have no idea if I'll outlive my third and current husband. Yes, ladies, I remarried in my 60s after 27 years of being single to a man nine years older. He's probably not as healthy as I am and more overweight than I am so who knows which one of us will knock on the pearly gates first.

The fact is, there are many more baby boomer women than men alive today. Like most of those women, I like men even though I don't have a great track record when it comes to choosing the right one to marry. My current situation is the exception.

I still believe that women never lose their interest in finding a good man to enjoy spending some of their time with. A good man to talk to. Make decisions with. Sleep with. Appreciate the things he does better and enjoy the things that we women do better. As long as he doesn't smother me with too much togetherness, I definitely think being with someone you love is infinitely better than being alone. Being with someone you can't stand? Forget it. In that case, the single life is the best life. So, our goal, then, is to find the right guy. Hopefully, this is the book that will help with that. Lord knows I've had plenty of experience.

Some people might think I either don't understand men or I'm not that comfortable around them. To my way of thinking, though, the fact that I've been married, divorced and annulled twice, and am currently on my third and hopefully my last marriage is proof enough that I have, at the very least, learned some helpful lessons about men over the years. Before this last time at the altar, I also wove my way in and out of two reasonably serious relationships. One lasted eight months, the other two-and-a-half years. Then, for 11 years I didn't date anyone. I just worked to get my kids through college.

I'm the first to admit that when it comes to certain things, I don't have a clue to understanding men. The following might be a lame example, but I hope it will at least help explain the big difference between how some men think versus how I think. The task is a simple autumn activity: getting rid of leaves. Here's how I did it when I owned my own house with a 120x100-foot yard and at least 25 towering trees. First, I'd turn on my mulcher mower, mow the yard, and pulverize the leaves into smithereens, providing natural fertilizer for the grass. Then, I'd return the mower to the garage and enjoy a good book.

But that's not the way I've seen many men do it. Having observed my dad, brother, uncles, cousins, ex-husbands, neighbors, and friends in their annual effort to get rid of leaves, here is how many of the men I've known approach this project. First, they buy a full-size John Deere lawn tractor with an 8-foot blade for grass cutting. Then, they buy a rider mower for tight spaces and a regular lawn mower for really tight spaces. After that, they fabricate a huge round leaf blower that also sucks up leaves, and they attach that to the rider mower. Their next purchase is a wagon to pull behind the rider mower to catch the leaves from the blower. They drive around the yard on the rider mower, sucking up leaves and blowing them into the huge wagon. Next, they dump the leaves in the corner of the yard and bag them into huge plastic bags, after which they distribute them to various trees and shrubs for mulch. When a giant wind blows them all over yard again, they repeat the four previous steps. Then, they climb onto their full-size John Deere tractor after attaching a new front-end loader to lift the bags of leaves to another part of the yard behind the shed so the neighbors can't see the bags. Then, a few months after that, using the front-end loader again, they bring the bags of leaves to the garage area where a new $1500 stick-and-leaf mulcher machine now resides, a machine that puts out 85,000 decibels of noise with each operation. They take the leaves out of the bags and carefully dump each bag into the new $1500 stick-and-leaf mulcher

Patricia Lorenz

contraption. Finally, they take the mulched-up leaves and dump them into the new spreader attached to the full-size John Deere tractor and distribute them evenly around the yard to provide natural fertilizer.

It's a man thing. You gotta love a guy who will go to all that trouble. Think of the exercise he's getting, of his communing with nature, and his solving one little problem after another. Beats being a couch potato with a bag of Ruffles under each arm. But do you see my point? Men are totally different creatures than women and, come on, it's not easy finding the right one to look at in the wee hours of the morning and say goodnight to late at night with a smile on your face, especially at my (our) age. I assume if you're reading this book you're in your 40s, 50s, 60s, 70s, 80s or 90s.

The truth is that I truly enjoy being around men. For a married woman, I do have many male friends: old ones, young ones, and middle-agers. Most of them are happily married, young enough to be my sons, priests, or married to my women friends. In other words, off limits. That's why I like them so much. No sexual tension. Just interesting guy talk. I like to talk to men about everything from politics to religion, from projects in the garage to jokes they hear at work, from "what's wrong with the sump pump" to "let me tell you how to haggle with a used car salesman." I love to talk to men about school work, housework, woodwork, books, movies, landscaping, terrorism, and the state of the Union. I like to watch football with men.

For ten years, before I moved to Florida in 2004, I ran a crash pad in my home in Milwaukee for airline pilots. I had an empty nest and three extra bedrooms so often I'd have two, three, four, or maybe even five happily married airline pilots using the extra bedrooms in my house as their local crash pad. They all lived in other states but needed a place

4

to crash in Milwaukee because they were all employees of Midwest Airlines, based at Milwaukee's international airport. Since I lived seven minutes from the airport, it was a perfect arrangement. Snow White and the seven dwarfs.

Imagine kibitzing with different men off and on during every week of the year. Men who treat you with respect because they're a guest in your home. Men who make you laugh, fix things around the house, and clean up after themselves, including their own bathroom. Imagine having one or two good-looking, funny, handsome men hanging around your home, men who never, ever, ever, ever complained if I put a little dent in my car, smelled up the house with my garlic-infested cooking, or talked on the phone too much.

Indeed, my life as a single woman during those ten years that I ran the crash pad was downright joyful, thanks to those male pilots. Those men spoiled me when it came to looking for and dating men when I moved to Florida, that's for sure. But I'm also sure that observing those 40 or so men who stayed in my crash pad during those ten years was very helpful when it came to choosing my third, and hopefully my final, husband.

So, yes, there's a big difference in the way men and women do things, think, react, solve problems, tackle projects, and communicate. Sometimes, the difference is unbelievable (see above leaf-removal example), and sometimes it's downright exasperating. Most of the time, though, the difference is marvelous. Thought-provoking. For me, anyway, it seems that as the years go by, it gets easier and easier to make friends with men. Because of that fact, my life is unbelievably interesting and happy.

However, this book is not just about how perfectly wonderful it is to be with a man. It's about struggles, finding dates, enduring the long, long time it takes to get to know a man and deciding if you really, truly want to put up with their weird way of doing things in exchange for the truly amazing things about them that we women cherish. This book is about the good, the bad, the ugly, the cheap, the generous, the faithless, the blessed, the angry, the insecure, the positive, and the negative—true stories about various men who have crossed my path. This book is about getting-to-know-you conversations, adventures, and experiences with the men I've met, dated, admired, and banished (often after one date) in order to maintain my sense of happiness and self-worth so that you, too, can go down this path better informed.

Whether your dream is to find Mr. Perfect and get married or just to have a male friend and/or lover as your full-time companion, I hope and pray this book helps you do just that. The thing is, the older we get, the harder it is to find the right person. It's also hard to decide if we middle-aged and older women even want to share our lives again with a man.

Sometimes, our children put a big kink in our plans. I have a friend whose father, a widower, remarried. My friend was dead-set against the marriage and now finds that her stepmother is in her own words, "Absolutely awful! She makes me feel like an outsider in my father's house. She wants my father all to herself and even had the nerve to get rid of some of Mother's furniture and linens."

Every time I see this woman she has more and more complaints about her stepmother. One time she was upset that her dad and her stepmother were spending two or three months in Florida every winter.

Funny thing though, whenever I see her dad and stepmom, they seem to be deliriously happy. The daughter is the only one who's miserable, wallowing in her selfishness, making herself unhappier every year.

Let me tell you about my own dad's remarriage. In 1979, when I was pregnant with my youngest child, my mother died at age 57, in the prime of her life, of ALS. My mother was my best friend, and her death devastated me. Three years later, my Dad remarried. I'd only been with Bev a couple of times before the wedding, but each time I could tell how happy she and my Dad were together. I admit that I wondered how it would feel to have another woman living in the house my Dad built in 1947, the house that we children grew up in and that my mother had lovingly decorated all those years we were growing up. How would it feel to have another woman in Mother's home?

Even though I loved my mother deeply, I honestly believe an angel was sitting on Dad's shoulder when he met, dated, and married Bev. During the early years of their marriage, that same angel sat on my shoulder, reminding me to keep an open mind about my dad's new love.

Since their marriage I've seen firsthand that Bev is a gem, a beautiful human being whose optimistic personality and ready-to-do-anything-or-go-anywhere attitude add sparkle to my Dad's life. Together, they have traveled the country by car or plane, visiting Dad's friends and relatives or going to his World War II reunions or antique car club get-togethers. Bev has just smiled and loved every minute of their adventures.

Over the years they redecorated nearly every room in the house. Thanks to Bev's beautiful taste, the home of my childhood is lovelier today than it was when I was growing up.

Three months after they were married Dad had a heart attack. Lovingly, Bev nursed him back to health and encouraged him to go walking or biking with her every day. They went dancing many Saturday nights, traveled the world together, and entertained their many combined friends and relatives.

Bev even understands how important it is for Dad to have plenty of time to putter out in the barn on his many projects. She likes to putter inside the house while he's in the barn so, like Jack Sprat and his wife, they get along fine.

In all the years of their marriage since 1982, I've never heard Dad and Bev have a serious argument. Oh, they tease each other every once in a while, but never sarcastically. They respect each other, and both seem completely happy and content with their lives as they enjoy their golden years together.

I don't even like to think about what life could have been like for my Dad all these years if he'd never met or married Bev. I honestly believe he'd be a sad, lonely, old man. Instead, because he had the courage in his 60s to move his life forward with a new woman and new love, he's a vibrant, healthy old codger who's as delightful and interesting as he is happy.

In 2015 when Dad was 95 and Bev 90 they both joined the YMCA and began to work out three times a week. After an hour of treadmill and exercise machines, they go out for lunch then home for a nap. What a life!

Over the years, I've gotten to know my stepmother increasingly better and realize she's the best thing that could have ever happened to Dad after Mom's death. I've also discovered that I'd truly like her as a person even if she weren't married to my Dad. When I visit them in Illinois, she and I often spend more time together than Dad and I do.

These middle-and-older-years second marriages remind me of the miracle of the wine at the marriage feast of Cana. When the couple ran out of wine, Jesus turned water into wine. One of the servants exclaimed. "Master, you saved the best for last."

In the marriage feast, I think the good Lord often does save the best times for last even when it means starting over with a new spouse. I know one thing for sure. I'm just glad the good Lord gave me the courage to tuck the warm, wonderful memories I have of my own mother into the bottom of my heart and to allow the good, new feelings I have for my stepmother to blossom and flourish. I've learned that if we just open our hearts and minds to change, life seems to get better as we get older. I know it has for my Dad, thanks to Bev. Moreover, my father's remarriage has taught me that finding a good man in midlife and beyond is not only possible but quite probable if we women just keep our wits about us during the dating process.

I pray this book will offer encouragement for women who need a little push to get back on the bicycle after someone breaks your heart or a spouse dies. Believe me, my heart has been ripped to sharp little shards by a number of men who have stepped across the line and into my heart and psyche and then torn it every which way but healthy. I will share the pain with you. I will also share how I survived and moved on.

A good, healthy, happy relationship between a man and a woman is a precious, much sought-after gift. But it takes work. Lots and lots and lots and lots of work. Let me share what I've experienced and learned, and then prayerfully you'll be able to get busy and open your heart to finding a man you, too, can cherish and be happy with. Did I mention it takes lots and lots and lots of work?

Patricia Lorenz

1

Sam, First Husband

I'm writing this book for women in their 40s, 50s, 60s, 70s, 80s and 90s who are single, divorced, or widowed and who are interested in finding a good man with whom to share the rest of their lives. In order to do that I must first unzip my soul and expose my foibles. Think about it. Nobody wants to read about the perfect woman in the perfect house wearing the perfect designer outfit with the perfect man at her side. We women want the real belly-in-the-muck-of-life story. We want to read about the tough parts, the sad, anguishing parts of a real woman's life, and hopefully learn how she wiggled out of the mud and muck into the light with a pretty good man's arms available for a great bear hug every so often. So, that's what I'm going to give you. The truth.

I've made many mistakes when it comes to men, but I don't think I'm that much different from many women. After all, the divorce rate is inching toward 60% in this country and perhaps the world. The "until death do us part" section of the marriage vows doesn't seem to hold any water these days because our containers all have holes in them.

That said, permit me to share my earlier, more youthful experiences with the men in my life. I was 22 years old when I married my first husband. Way, way, way too young. I know this now. But then? My excuse is that nobody is wise at 22. Back then, birth control methods weren't nearly as sophisticated or as accurate. If I'd had the wisdom at that young age that I have now, I wouldn't be writing this book, and I wouldn't have had such an interesting life filled with so many struggles, relationship experiences, and adventures. I count all my struggles as blessings, by the way. That's what happens when you get older. I'm older and have a lot to look back on.

So, let's take a step back to 1968 when I was fresh out of college and had just moved to Denver, Colorado by myself to start my first big adventure. I chose Denver because my college boyfriend Sam offered to let me live in his Denver apartment rent-free for three months. He was being sent to Houston for classes during that time for the company that had just hired him.

When the three months ended and Sam returned, we celebrated a little too much. When the urine test came back positive, my only hope for salvation was not telling my parents who lived in Illinois. In high school, three of my first cousins got pregnant out of wedlock in one year's time, and my father was furious. I remember distinctly when he said "If you ever get pregnant before marriage, don't think for a minute that you can come running home and we'll take care of everything. You sleep in the bed you make." So, when the unthinkable happened, I knew I had to solve the dilemma myself with the help of my boyfriend Sam, the guy whose thesis I'd typed when he was working on his master's degree in geology at Southern Illinois University where I was finishing up my bachelor's degree.

Sam had moved to Denver a few months before I did, and when my pregnancy test came back positive Sam was more than willing to get married since he'd had that in mind all along. I was still worried about his daily drinking habits, and the thought of marrying him was pretty far down on the list for me. Being pregnant, though, scared me to death. Being an unwed mother back in the 60s was a much bigger deal than it is today; that's for sure.

I knew Sam had marriage to me in mind before we left college when one night as I was perched on the single step leading into the mobile home I shared with three other co-eds, he looked into my eyes and out of the blue said, "Will you nurse our babies when we have them?" Since my ta-tas were practically at his eye level (remember, I was standing on a step) he must have been distracted enough to pop such a question. At the time, I didn't find it particularly amusing. I hadn't even considered getting married, much less to him.

But there I was a year later, pregnant, determined not to tell my folks, and scared to go back home to Illinois. I was at the mercy of the father of my child. Neither Sam nor I were big on lavish weddings, so we planned an atrocity of a wedding in about 15 minutes.

Both of us were hard at work at our first real better-than-minimum-wage jobs. Neither of us had vacation time coming. Neither of us had any relatives in the state of Colorado. We certainly didn't have the money to spend on a big wedding.

So, a few days later in June 1968, a day I remember being filled with anguish, fear, and embarrassment, mostly on my part, we both simply said, "Let's do it." And we did. There were 13 of us in the tiny chapel. Later, we all went out to our favorite hang-out, drank margaritas, and ate popcorn to celebrate our nuptials. When I look back on it, I think the wedding and the reception afterward may have had something to do with the state of the honeymoon. The state of the honeymoon may have had a lot to do with the demise of the marriage a few years later.

Ah, yes...the honeymoon! We both managed to get Monday off, and since the wedding was on Friday night, we had three days. The groom, being a geologist, a man who loved rocks and strange natural formations and earthly oc-currences, announced after the wedding that we were go-ing to drive to Yellowstone National Park, over 400 miles away. That man loved to drive, but I wasn't very sure about spending the bulk of my three-day honeymoon cooped up in a car. Getting there and back would take two full days which only left us a day to enjoy Yellowstone, but this was back in the 60s when men still got their way about almost everything.

So, we drove. And drove. We'd jump out of the car, eat a fast meal, and get right back in the car. I oohed and aahed at the incredible scenery that whizzed by at 75, sometimes 80, miles per hour. When we reached snow drifts that were eight feet tall in northern Wyoming, he paused for five minutes to take my picture next to them. I stood there in my sleeveless blouse and summer-weight slacks in early June and made a snowball to throw at my groom.

Back in the car we drove for hours, winding our way through mountainous roads toward Yellowstone. We ar-rived at dark and spent the night in a primitive, cold cabin. I stayed awake much of the night, worrying about bears. By noon Sunday, after a huge brunch loaded with mountain man eggs, sausage, and pancakes the size of plates, I began to feel awful. I thought back to the week before the wed-ding and realized I'd been constipated for an entire week.

The quickness of the wedding, worrying about taking a day off work from my new job, irregular meals, perhaps a little morning sickness, and spending eleven hours in the car the day before had blocked me up completely.

By the time we finally arrived at the peak look-out-point of the entire honeymoon, the Old Faithful geyser, I was one miserable 22-year-old bride. As I sat on a long wooden bench with a couple dozen other "Old Faithful" watchers waiting for the spectacle, I felt as if I was carrying the weight of the world in my gut. Misery was my middle name as I watched my new husband pacing back and forth, waiting anxiously for his geological wonder to blow.

This is my honeymoon, for heaven's sake! I can't let this go on, I thought to myself.

Holding my stomach in pain, I swallowed my shyness and gathered my courage. "Sam, I need some prune juice. Would you mind going in to the camp store to see if they have any?"

My groom, who wasn't too crazy about the possibility of missing the start of Old Faithful's show, dashed into the store and returned in record time, handing me a quart of room temperature prune juice. "Here. You'll have to drink it from the bottle," he snorted.

As we sat there waiting for the explosion of one of the world's greatest natural wonders, I drank my juice. We waited, and I drank. Suddenly, the geyser put on its show, spewing hot steam hundreds of feet into the air. I watched and drank my prune juice, wishing my innards could spew like that geyser.

After the show, we climbed back into the car for a driving tour of the enormous national park. When a bear cub ambled across the road and climbed up to the window of the car in front of us, I snapped a quick photo, finished off my quart of prune juice, and wished I was back home in a nice tub of hot water, easing my intestinal pains.

As we neared the park exit later that afternoon after a long, long drive through Yellowstone's immensity, Mother Nature and the prune juice grabbed hold of my stopped-up digestive system and started the rumblings of a geyser in my gut that felt as if it would rival that of Old Faithful.

"Sam! You have to find a bathroom! I have to go! Now! Please, get to a bathroom! Hurry!"

My groom sped up for half-a-mile, then slammed on the brakes. "It's up there." He pointed to a thick, dense forested area.

"Up where?" I started to panic. I didn't see anything but a huge hill and thousands of trees.

"Right there, off to the right. See that building? It's an outhouse."

I shot my husband a look that could have caused flowers to wilt and slammed the car door as I bolted out. I stumbled up the steep hill and dashed toward the outhouse, noting that it was much darker up there in the forest. The sun was starting to go down, and the shadows were ominous.

"There better be lights in this place," I mumbled to myself.

It was a two-seater outhouse. No lights. No toilet paper. No nothing, except two smelly holes and spider webs all over the place. But at that moment as Mother Nature's grip on my intestines catapulted my mind back to reality, I plopped my quickly exposed bare fanny on hole number one. One explosion after another punctuated the silence in the woods as I prayed that my new husband had the car windows rolled up so he couldn't hear what I was up to up there in the woodland privy. I sat there in that smelly pit, terrorized that a bear or a snake would amble in while I was going about my business.

An hour later, after having lost approximately ten pounds, I staggered out the door, holding my slacks in front of me. "Sam," I hollered weakly, "Could you bring some tissues up here?" At that moment, I could have killed for a roll of toilet paper.

All he could find were a couple paper napkins from the last fast-food restaurant we'd visited. I used every square inch of those napkins and then prayed that we'd get to our hotel quickly.

That night the prune juice continued its onslaught, having realized it had to do a week's worth of work in just a day. Inside our hotel room, I quickly made a dash for the bathroom. My husband plopped down on the bed after adjusting the TV set that was hooked to the wall up near the ceiling. After an hour of percussion noises that radiated from the bathroom, he peeked in the door and said, "Hey, darlin', I know you don't feel too good, but how would it be if I adjust this TV so you can see it from in here? If you leave the door open, you can watch from in the bathroom and I can watch it from the bed. At least, you won't be so lonely." After that, he poured himself another big glass of Kessler's whiskey, his nightly drink of choice, then proceeded to watch some godawfulboring fishing show.

Embarrassment, disgust, and misery punctuated the rest of my evening and continued well into the night as I sat there on the Motel 6 toilet, watching bad TV, as my husband spent the night alone in the bed on the other side of the bathroom wall. *Welcome to the real world of marriage,* I thought to myself as the sounds and smells radiating from my body began to cool down. As I gently fondled the huge, soft roll of toilet paper before me, I actually said prayers of thanksgiving to the Almighty for that little bit of paradise—that nice, shiny white bathroom where I spent the third and final night of my honeymoon.

Life with Sam was not one big giant trip to a national park, believe me. I quickly learned that he liked booze better than me. That man seemed to live on vodka and whiskey. I remember the day I figured out he was spending more than 10% of our monthly income on booze. The man was tithing alcohol, and I felt cheated, compromised, and foolish as his wife. I haven't even gotten to the part about the physical abuse yet.

In 1970, nearly a year after our first child was born, Sam and I had been looking for a house to buy so we could move from the small apartment we'd rented in Denver. One day he came home from work early.

"Pat, I have to tell you something," he said with his usual southern Illinois twang.

"Wait, I have great news!" I interrupted him. "I just talked to the realtor. Our loan was approved. We got the house! The closing's in two weeks, and we can move in the next day!"

"Pat, there isn't going to be any house. I just got laid off at work. We're going to be leaving Denver."

I couldn't speak. Our dream house, the red brick bungalow with the built-in bookcases on each side of the fireplace and built-in buffet in the dining room, was everything I had always wanted in a home. My husband and I had spent months looking for this, our first house. Jeanne, our baby, was just a year old. The house was two blocks from a beautiful park with a lake and flower-lined meandering paths, perfect for a mom pushing a stroller.

In spite of my frantic prayers for a quick solution to this disaster, we had to leave our beloved Colorado mountains to start over in Missouri, where my husband secured a teaching job at a junior college.

Two weeks after arriving in Kirkwood, Missouri, I discovered that I was expecting another child. Meanwhile, I unpacked in our new apartment while my husband settled into his new teaching position. This apartment had two huge bedrooms, central air, and even a pool and play area out back. I rekindled a close friendship with one of my favorite cousins who lived in the area, and before long, starting over didn't seem so bad after all.

In January 1971, Julia bounced into the world. Seventeen months later, in May 1972, after buying our first home, a tiny brick bungalow with a huge back yard, we welcomed Michael into the world. Both conceptions had involved heavy drinking on Sam's part and, more often than not, physical coercion on his part even to get me into the same bed with him. Fertility should have been my middle name.

With three children less than four years old and a husband who drank 3/4 of a quart bottle of booze every night of his life, our lives fell apart completely. Extreme unhappiness, frequent abuse, and a sense of fear forced me to seek advice from my pastor who suggested that divorce might be the only answer. I did everything I could to hold things together, but friends, family, neighbors, counselors, and even my pastor advised me to end the marriage and start over.

On November 13, 1975, after driving from northern Illinois to St. Louis, Missouri, then spending most of the day in divorce court with me, my mother and father helped load the moving truck. That evening my folks, my three children—ages three, four and six—and I left Missouri, crossed the Mississippi River, and drove up through the state of Illinois to my hometown of Rock Falls, Illinois.

I'll never forget the first piece of mail I received at our new home, a 98-year-old rented frame house. I quickly tore open the envelope.

Patricia Lorenz

November 17, 1975

My dearest Patricia,

This little communiqué hopefully will be the first one arriving at your new home. Welcome home!

For a little while Thursday evening while I was wheeling that big U-Haul eastward over the Mississippi, I felt like Moses leading his flock out of bondage.

A great burden has been lifted from our minds now knowing you are free from further abuse. We felt almost helpless to do anything before. Thank God, that is all past now.

Lovingly,

Dad

Thus began my life as a single parent and the end of my first real relationship with a man. The number one thing I learned from that entire 8-year experience (from meeting Sam in college to divorcing him in 1975) is that alcohol is a killer. Alcohol kills love, relationships, happiness, parenting skills, and any hope for a normal life. I pray that you will reread that last sentence many, many times. Write it down. *Alcohol kills love, relationships, happiness, parenting skills, and any hope for a normal life.*

Harold, Second Husband

My first stint at single parenthood began near the love and support of my parents who were into their 30th year of a happy marriage.

"Mom, this old house is wonderful!" I gushed. "The children love their new backyard, the swinging gate, and climbing trees. The neighbor kids are flocking in from all sides."

The next month I found an interesting job at a radio station, and starting over wasn't nearly as scary as I thought it would be. In fact, that time was the best time of my life.

A year later when I was broadcasting a parade for the radio station, I met a man who had come from Wisconsin to judge the high school band parade competition. Even though my mother warned me about the 17-year difference in our ages, Harold and I continued to see each other every weekend for the next two years.

When Harold started talking about getting married, I wasn't sure I was ready to start over again in another marriage, especially in another state with a much older man who had six children and was already a grandpa, but Harold was quite persuasive.

Just four months before our wedding, however, my mother, who in recent years had become my best friend, was diagnosed with Lou Gehrig's disease, ALS. I simply couldn't move to another state and leave my parents. I wanted to spend as much time as possible with my mother so I talked Harold into trying to find a job in our little town of Rock Falls, Illinois instead of the children and me moving to Wisconsin to his town.

Trouble is, he had just changed jobs from being the high school band director to being the assistant principal. Even though he tried, he couldn't find a job anywhere in northern Illinois that came close to his salary in Wisconsin. So, Harold and I got married in Rock Falls, Illinois, and the children and I stayed there while Harold commuted on weekends. For almost 2 1/2 years after we were married, he left the high school in Wisconsin at 4 p.m. every Friday and drove the three hours to our home in Illinois. Then, every Monday morning he got up at 4 a.m. so he could drive back to Wisconsin, arriving at the school by 7:30am.

Unfortunately, during that time my beloved mother died from ALS. Harold and I were expecting a baby by then, which was another shock, considering the fact that Harold was in his 50's and his six kids and six grandchildren seemed to be quite enough for this man who was already dreaming of retirement. Harold was a trooper, though, and actually passed out cigars to his friends the day he learned I was pregnant. Andrew was born in the December following my mother's death on August 1st, 1979.

So, there I was, married to my second husband, the man I only saw on weekends, and raising four children alone in Illinois during the weekdays. It was a strange arrangement. I have to say Harold made the best of it. He never complained about the 3-hour each way commute. During the week, he spent his free time baking so he could bring his special breads to the children and me. He even won some blue ribbons at the state fair with his cranberry bread and zucchini nut bread.

Harold taught me a lot about the sacrifices ones makes to make a marriage work. To this day, I still treasure the fact that Harold agreed to let me and the children live in my hometown where my parents were during those horrible months when mother was dying of ALS.

Ten months after Andrew was born, Harold insisted that the children and I move to Wisconsin so he could stop his weekend commute. I certainly understood Harold's need to have his new immediate family close at hand so I agreed to the move.

Starting over this time was the hardest I'd ever done: while still grieving for my mother, I had to uproot and move four children, sell a house, leave behind a great job at the local radio station, and say goodbye to a host of friends and relatives. On Halloween day in a caravan of cars and a rental truck, the four children and I headed north to Wisconsin.

"Six bedrooms, a big yard, lots of trees? Harold, the house is perfect!" I was thrilled when I saw our new home. The children thrived in their new school. I found a part-time job at another radio station. The neighbors were nice. Harold was happy that he didn't have to commute anymore, and we all loved our new, sprawling home.

We lived happily ever after, right? Not quite. I quickly learned that this older man I'd married did not thrive in a household with three preteens and a baby. The stress of our new blended family, including Harold's six grown children, in-laws, and six grandchildren from his previous marriage, was a bit different from the carefree fun and romance we'd enjoyed on the weekends for the past three years when Harold was still making the weekly trek to our home in Illinois.

The next five years of our marriage were a roller coaster experience. One minute it was Camelot, the next minute unbearable. Before long the unbearable times were the norm, and I suggested we separate for a year to figure out and solve our problems without the everyday stresses eating at us.

One Sunday afternoon Harold and I sat down and mapped out a plan for an amicable separation that we agreed would only last a year. We both hoped it would give us enough time to figure out how to make the marriage work.

Harold moved into a nice apartment just three miles from our home where he could have peace and quiet and not be bombarded by the preschool, middle-school and high-school set. We visited each other often, went on a few dates, and made arrangements for some serious marriage counseling.

Two months after we separated, when I thought everything was going great and was about to suggest another appointment with a marriage counselor, a stranger came to the door and served me with divorce papers.

"Harold!" I practically hollered into the phone, "We need more time! Why are you doing this?" I was shocked that he wanted to end it so suddenly and completely.

"It's over," he said firmly. "I want a divorce."

Not again. I just couldn't start over again. Not with four children and a two-day-a-week job. But this time I had 15 years' worth of starting overs under my belt. I'd not only survived each one, but somehow each new start had brought wonderful people and experiences into our lives. Somehow, I got through those months of turmoil and hurt.

The day our divorce was final, Harold married the woman he'd been dating for months. She was a divorced woman closer to his own age who'd never had any children. Perhaps Harold needed a simpler life than what I could offer.

Within a month my part-time job at the radio station became a four-day-a-week career. With the help of child support for Andrew, some extra writing jobs, and the various jobs my teenagers had, we were able to keep going financially and stay in the house we'd all grown to love.

The children and I laughed and cried together, spilt milk without any fog-like tension at the dinner table, created adventures for ourselves, made a home for each other, and figured out ways to get the three oldest through college at the same time.

Harold died of leukemia in 1989, just two years after he remarried. Andrew, the son he and I had together, was nine years old at the time of his father's death. Once again, our lives took on a starting-over feeling. Although I wondered if I could raise Andrew alone, without the benefit of his father's love and guidance, I knew it could be done. After all, I'd learned something many years before in Denver, Colorado when my dream house evaporated and I had to start over in a new state with my first husband. I'd learned that starting over after a divorce or in a new job, a new town, a different financial situation, with a new spouse, or after the death of someone you love almost always leads to something better—if you put your trust in God and just bulldoze ahead. I also learned that women are strong and that marriage is very, very hard.

Patricia Lorenz

3

Mom's Got a Date Tonight

When you're used to sharing your life with someone, to be suddenly single can be the most devastating, lonely, life-shaking experience in the world. Just ask any separated, divorced or widowed person. The thought of starting over in a new relationship, though, is the most terrifying thing you can imagine.

In 1987 when my divorce was final after a two-year separation, my four children had different ideas. After a couple years of being my dates at movies and fast food restaurants, I heard comments like, "Mom, why don't you join that singles group at church and meet some men?"

I shot back, "I don't know how to meet men or go out on dates. Besides, who wants a 40-year-old woman with four kids and a big mortgage?"

But the children kept after me to do something for myself, and so I worked up my nerve and joined the *Single Again* group at church. A few weeks later, the entire membership went out for a fish fry and dancing afterward. Twenty-one women and one man. That poor guy danced with every one of us, bless his heart. When the dance was over, he sort of limped out the door, alone.

I whined to my friends, "I think fish sticks at home would have been more fun than waiting for my turn with Mr. Trip-the-Light-Fantastic."

For the next few months, I kept my social calendar filled by attending my son's high school basketball games, watching Julia cheerlead, attending Jeanne's piano recitals, getting more involved at church, and treating myself to an occasional dinner out with other single women friends.

Then, one day it happened. A man who advertised on the radio station where I worked invited me out to dinner. I was terrified, and my children knew it. Julia beamed, "Mom, he's probably really cute and maybe even rich. Maybe he'll take you to a really nice restaurant."

Well, he was rich, all right. Too rich. He not only took me to a very nice restaurant, he mentioned that he owned the place and that it was a tax write-off for one of the state's biggest companies that he also owned. He'd just returned from South America on an art-buying expedition and was eager to take me to his penthouse to show me his antiques. Okay, I can see you howling and slapping your knee. I know it sounds fishy, straight out of a B movie. But it's all true. He did own the restaurant and was really super rich, something that was so far from my reality that I honestly didn't know how to say "no" to the guy when he insisted he show me his digs, but I worked up my courage and told him a big lie—that I didn't like antiques. No way was I going to this geezer's condo even if it was enormous and on a lake. Believe me, a woman who had to struggle all afternoon to find one decent going-out-to-dinner outfit midst her suburban wardrobe of jeans and jogging clothes, had no business with a rich tycoon twenty years her senior who celebrated every other topic of conversation with another drink.

"Lord, I'm sorry about the lie. I really do like antiques," I whispered aloud as I drove myself home when the date was over.

At home that night, Jeanne was waiting up for me. "So, Mom, tell me all about him. Did you have fun?"

I took a deep breath. "Honey, he was just too old, too rich, and drank too much to suit my tastes."

"Mother, you're never going to find a man with that attitude," Jeanne quipped.

I prayed a lot that night. "Okay, Lord, I need a little help here. I'm not really looking for a man, am I? Don't I have enough to do with my life without complicating it with another adult? I'm just getting used to the idea of being *head of household*, and I rather like the responsibility. You were proud of me, weren't you, when I learned to use an axe to split wood for the wood burner? When I revved up the chain saw to cut the wood down to size, I felt like Paul Bunyan, but after a weekend of wood splitting and sawing, I don't have the energy to smile politely, let alone look for a date. Amen."

A year later, after putting over 15,000 miles on my little car running the kids all over kingdom come with their myriad of activities, it happened again. My second date.

This gentleman owned an advertising agency, and we went out under the guise of my doing some copywriting work for him. We didn't talk much business during dinner, but when the check came and I offered to help pay, he pointed out that the meal was tax deductible. I didn't feel much like a date after that, but the real clincher as to why I never went out with him again was the fact that the entire conversation centered on his two passions in life: golf and tennis. For a woman who has never picked up a club or a racket, it was a real *D&B* night. Dull and boring.

When I reported to my kids about that fiasco, Jeanne replied, "Mom, that's what you said about your date last year. You're too picky. Do you like being single?"

"So, what's wrong with being single? Just because I spent most of my adult years being married doesn't mean I can't re-adjust, does it?"

During the next year, my social life got busier, without any more dates, I might add. I ushered for a few musicals at a Milwaukee theater with another single mother, then watched the performances on the house. I joined the education committee at church. I did some volunteer writing for a local singles magazine. Andrew, my youngest, and I made new friends when we joined a single parents and children's group that met for dinner and a discussion every week. On Fridays, we watched Michael play basketball and Julia cheerlead. On Saturdays, we rented movies, popped popcorn, and relaxed at home.

The next year another friend called. "You have to meet Ben. He's single, your age, no kids, and wants to meet someone who likes quiet evenings at home watching movies on TV. He doesn't go out much, but he's very good about fixing things around the house. You might like him."

Like him because he's a handyman? What sort of personality trait is that? I wondered if Mary decided to go out with Joseph because he was handy with wood. "Well, at least maybe this guy can fix my snow blower," I thought to myself.

Ben came over early one Saturday afternoon. We talked for a couple of hours. I could tell right away he wasn't someone I wanted to spend any more time with. Rather than waste his time I explained that I had to run some errands. He said, "I'll come with you, and then we'll rent a movie to watch later on."

I sputtered a bit and then muttered something like, "Well, if that's what you really want to do."

I asked myself, *Why am I so wishy-washy? I can't even say "no" to someone I know isn't Mr. Right.*

Just as the movie began, my children started coming home: Julia from her baby-sitting job, Andrew from visiting some friends, and Michael from his job at a local pharmacy. So, there we were in the family room. Me, in my big green rocker next to the wood burner, Ben on the couch next to my chair, Andrew next to Ben, and Julie next to Andrew. Michael plopped down on the love seat. A few minutes later, Tony and John, Michael's friends, came over and they squeezed in on the couch and the loveseat.

Well, now wasn't this cozy? Mom, her date, 8-year-old Andrew, and four teenagers. Michael kept looking at me sort of funny, like, "Where did you find this one, Mom?" I felt like I was on trial. Ben stood up, rubbed his slicked-back hair, and went over to investigate the innards of the wood burner again. He liked that contraption obviously more than he liked being in a room full of jovial teens, a full-of-energy second grader, and a woman who yawned a lot.

I wondered what the children thought of him, and I secretly wished he'd go home so I could put on my lounging pajamas and get comfortable. I wanted to read the paper and write a letter to my folks. Instead, I had to sit there and entertain this humorless gentleman who was probably thinking to himself that he hadn't expected a crowd when he asked if he could come over to get acquainted.

I closed my eyes for a second and prayed, "Lord, I know my friends and I have been grumbling about my meeting a nice man for years. Here's one sitting in my family room, and I can hardly wait until he goes home. Why am I so fickle? Do I really need or want to find someone special and get married again?"

These thoughts kept flitting through my head the entire eight hours and 20 minutes Ben stayed at our house that Saturday. When he finally left at midnight, I had to admit that being with someone for the wrong reasons is a lot worse than not being with anyone at all.

When I crawled into bed that night I thought to myself, *All right. I know I'm not ready to settle down again. I have four kids to finish raising. I'm already settled. Besides, I like who I am. The man of my dreams, the one who's easygoing, sensitive, intelligent, interesting, has a great sense of humor and a deep faith, just hasn't come around yet. Maybe he never will. That's okay. I feel like there's a light burning inside me that's all mine. My light. The one that keeps reminding me who I really am.*

Being single made me feel radiant for years although I have to admit that for many years I still asked my friends to keep their eyes open for a good man, preferably a pilot who golfs. Why? Because I figured he'd be gone a lot and I'd still have time to let my own light shine through.

4

Dancing Lessons

I'd been a single parent of four for five years and I worried about everything. About whether the sump pump would conk out during a big rain and flood my family room when I wasn't home. About wasp's nests in the overhang and broken tree limbs in the gutter. About how I would put four kids through college, three at the same time. About how I would ever find a nice man to date and how sad it would be to grow old alone.

One Saturday evening the phone rang. It was a nice man with a deep voice telling me I'd won a free dance lesson.

"It's fun, and you'll learn lots of different dance steps," he proclaimed convincingly.

"It's really free?" I asked timidly.

"Absolutely!" the man gushed in the key of G. "It's just our way of introducing you to the wonderful world of dancing."

When I hung up the phone, I could feel my face flush. *What if I step on my instructor's toes and make a fool of myself?*

At class the following week, a woman dressed in a black chiffon skirt and red spangled *Wizard of Oz* high-heeled shoes glided toward me, followed by two 20-something young men. She reached for my hand. "Hello, there! I'm Ms. West, one of the instructors. This is Mr. Bates. And here's Mr. Ross. We only use last names here to keep it formal. Ballroom dancing, you know, is very serious."

"Serious?" I gasped. These were not serious people. With giant grins etched onto their faces and their happy feet tip-tapping around the dance floor, they were bouncy, peppy, light-on-their-feet little gremlins. Definitely not serious. This was happy feet land.

"All right," one of the instructors called out cheerily. "Everyone join hands and make a big circle. We're going to do the 'push-pull.' Pretend you're squishing grapes. Right foot back, ladies, and squish! Now left foot forward and squish! Pretend you're marching in a parade. Right foot forward, flat on the floor, march! Left foot down, march! So, it's squish, squish, march, march."

I did it with the others. Squished my grapes, marched my parade. Squish, squish, march, march. Over and over.

Then, we had to do it with a partner. Mr. Ross, one of the most handsome of the half-my-age instructors, rushed over to take my hand. I felt my heart beating faster while Mr. Ross and I squish-squished and march-marched as I repeated the words over and over to myself with each beat of the music.

But then something awful happened. Mr. Ross started asking me questions—while we were push-pulling!

"So, how do you like dancing? And what do you do for a living?"

Two questions, and here I was trying desperately to keep my squish-squish, march-march in order. I could just feel what was about to happen. The minute I opened my mouth to answer, my squishes and marches got crossed. The smile never left his face when I stepped on his toes. "It's okay, Ms. Lorenz. We're going to teach you to do all this automatically so you'll look good on the dance floor. You'll learn the fox trot, waltz, rumba, jitterbug, mambo, cha-cha..."

All that in forty minutes? I wondered as I glanced at the large wall clock.

"Are you sure you've never had dance lessons before?" questioned the handsome one. "You're so light on your feet!"

Squish-squish. 'No, never did." *March-march.*

"So, what do you do?"

"I," *squish-squish,* "I'm a copywriter for a radio" *march-march* "station." *Squish-squish* "...write radio commercials." *March-march.*

"What do you do for fun? Are you married? Do you go dancing very often?"

All this from a man who refuses to tell me his first name? "Well, I don't do" *squish-squish* "much dancing socially, not married," *march-march,* "haven't danced for years, kinda rusty." *March-squish.* "Whoops! Sorry about that! By the way, my name's Pat."

Mr. Ballerina didn't flinch.

Finally, when the music ended, the instructors walked each guest, arm-in-arm to the other side of the room. It was time to watch the professionals put on a demonstration.

Poetry in motion. Straight out of the thirties. Arms a flying. Legs reaching for the sky. I could just see myself on the dance floor at my cousin's wedding, my heel up on my prince's shoulder for that split second while he twirled me so fast my full chiffon skirt would brush my cheek romantically before we ended our dance with his strong hands on my hips as he lifted me high above his head in a stunning spin finish. I was Ginger Rogers, and my partner was, ah, yes, Mr. Perfect.

Suddenly, Mr. Ross from the Happy Feet Gang, who looked like he hadn't yet had his fifth high-school reunion, stood before me and reached for my hand as if it were a paper-thin porcelain teacup. He carefully placed my hand upon his forearm as we glided ever-so-lightly onto the dance floor.

We squished, marched, waltzed, fox-trotted, and rumba'd. He kept asking me more personal questions while I tried desperately to keep my unhappy feet responding to his happy ones. I wondered if he were writing a book about my life.

After twenty-five minutes of squish-squish, march-march, question-question, talk about me but not about him, Mr. Ross ushered me into "The Room." I knew the minute he closed the door and the four dark floral-print wall-papered walls started to squeeze in on me that this was the place where they tried to force you to sign on the dotted line—the dotted line just under the part that said, "Ten one-hour lessons for $650, plus a $150 discount because you're such a swell, happy, light-on-your-feet person."

Mr. Ross started talking about my life, my social habits, my children, my lack of exercise, my need for more friends, my cash flow, the trouble I had meeting nice men, my career, my lonely Saturday nights, and my personal habits. He remembered every word I'd said. He talked and smiled. He flattered me. He made taking dancing lessons a synonym for turning my not-so-social life into a blaze of filled dance cards and stand-in-line gentlemen callers.

After reading a certificate on the wall over Mr. Ross's desk, I decided to change the focus of his inquisition by asking him why he'd gotten his master's degree in urban economics and was now a full-time dance instructor. As soon as the words were out of my mouth, Mr. Happy got happier. Every sentence he sputtered ended with an exclamation point.

"It's fun! Life is supposed to be fun! Dancing is fun! It's great exercise! It's a wonderful way to meet people! It's..." He went on for ten straight minutes, and I started to hate urban economics.

At last, he took a breath and touched my hand gently as he slid the contract under my fingers. His eyes sparkled. I felt his happy feet tapping under the desk.

I reached for the pen. On four lines of the contract, I wrote very slowly in neat, happy letters: "No money. Ain't funny. Too bad. So sad." Then, I stood up, smiled a happy smile, grabbed my coat, and bounded up the stairs toward the light.

A week later, I called some old friends and invited them to join me for a night on the town. After dinner we visited an old-fashioned '60s rock-and-roll club. We rocked, we rolled, we boogied, and we did The Twist. We laughed until our sides ached and danced until our legs gave out. We didn't do one squish-squish, march-march all night.

What I learned from Mr. Ross and the Happy Feet Gang is that it's up to me to make my life fun. Whether I'm 40, 50, 60, 70, or 80, in order to have friends, especially male friends, I must be a friend first. I have to make that first phone call and get things organized even if it means, heaven forbid, taking dancing lessons!

5

Tony:
The Relocated
Government Witness

By 1988, my oldest daughter had graduated from the Milwaukee High School of the Arts. Jeanne had been granted a year of study as a foreign exchange student in Yugoslavia thanks to a $1000 scholarship she received after winning the Junior Miss pageant in our hometown. My next two children, Julia and Michael, were both in high school, and Andrew was in grade school.

One thing I was looking forward to that year was the chance to teach writing at an enormous singles event called Single Fest, sponsored by the University of Wisconsin Milwaukee. A couple thousand singles from all over the Midwest would be attending various classes during the two days. After the classes, we'd all have a chance get to know each other at various dances and dinners in the evenings.

I taught my class one afternoon and was gathering up my materials to head for the banquet and one of the dances when a good-looking gentleman approached me.

"I'm looking for a writer, someone to help me write my book," he said as he flashed a big grin. He was dressed to the nines in a snazzy beige, almost off-white, summer suit. Few of the other participants were as dressed up so I paid attention, thinking, of course, *ah, this guy's cute, and he must be interesting if he thinks he's already had enough experiences to write a book.*

"Would you be interested in helping me write it?"

"What's it about? Why do you think your life is so interesting? You're not even 50 yet. You're not done living your life. Why don't you wait until you're older to write your memoir?"

"Let's talk about it at dinner. Will you join me?" Did I mention he was cute?

At dinner Tony told me he had just recently become a relocated government witness. He'd grown up in Brooklyn and had worked for the mob as a teen and into his 20's, even committed crimes for them. He couldn't become a made member of the mob, though, because he was only half Italian. To be a made member, you had to be full-blooded Italian. He told me about his crimes and about his interaction with various judges over the years. He talked about reform school. I was hooked. Interesting stuff, indeed.

As Tony rambled on about his life, I was trying to figure out when each week we could get together to write his book. Tony told me that in order to avoid prosecution for one of the crimes he'd committed for the mafia, the FBI convinced him to turn witness which meant he'd have to testify at some of the mob trials going on in New York. To protect him during that time they'd moved him to Milwaukee, Wisconsin, the land of cheese heads, beer, brats, bowling, Midwestern values, festivals, football, and fishing, far away from Brooklyn, Queens, and New York City.

That night Tony and I danced to our favorite rock and roll songs after dinner and began a 10-month relationship that involved a great friendship, including long talks about why I simply could not tolerate his racist attitudes. We made two trips to visit my dad and stepmom in Rock Falls, Illinois. One time down there, he and I were on the winning raft in the Rock River during the Raft Races that my dad organized.

Tony and I spent our Friday nights filled with dinners out, followed by cozy evenings in his small apartment in downtown Milwaukee. Then, he would follow me home to my big house in the suburbs where I allowed him to spend the night in my daughter Jeanne's room because that year she was in Yugoslavia as a foreign exchange student.

Every Saturday morning, we worked on the book in my home office. Together we wrote ten chapters. A book about Tony, a man who had used as many as five different last names in his life.

Imagine me, a 43-year-old mother of four, raised in a small town in northern Illinois, taught by nuns for 14 years, now single and being pursued by a very interesting man who wanted me to help him write his book! He seemed quite smitten with me as a woman as well, no doubt because opposites attract. Boy, were we opposite!

I was flattered, flustered, and flipping out of my mind over the fact that I was about to go out with a mafia wannabe who seemed like the nicest and most interesting guy in the world. I also loved the fact that he seemed to have much respect for my writing skills.

Before we started on the book I needed proof that Tony, with all his spine-tingling movie quality stories, was who he said he was. The proof was in a 29-page story in an old issue of *Life Magazine*. It was a special three-part section, titled "The Mob: Case History of a Gangland Murder."

It was a detailed account of the hit, the trial, and the verdict of the people vs. Sonny Franzese, Red Crabbe, Whitey Fiorio, and Tommy Matteo. Tony, the man in my life and book-writing partner, was one of the chief witnesses at that trial, and his name, his words at the trial, and his photo were plastered throughout the article. Four large photos of him, to be exact. The same man I was with only 20 years younger. Unmistakable. At least, I knew he wasn't giving me the biggest line of baloney in the dating world. Tony was definitely connected to the mob. I was hooked.

I insisted on keeping that copy of *Life Magazine* so I could prove to my friends and family that Tony was truly who he said he was. However, he didn't want any part of me telling anyone anything about him so he took the magazine back, much to my consternation. He didn't know that a few weeks later I found a different copy of that same magazine at a used bookstore at the Milwaukee airport in a section where they had hundreds of old issues of *Life Magazine*, organized by year and month. It was easy. I still have the magazine. It was all the proof I needed that I had befriended a wannabe member of a New York mob, a man who actually told the prosecuting attorney in the trial 20 years earlier that he always lied to the FBI because he had a lot to keep secret. Who would not want to help a man like that write the story of his life? I figured the stories themselves would be worth my time whether or not we ever finished or sold the book.

So, we began. Each Friday around 3 p.m., my normal time for leaving my job as copywriter at the radio station, I drove to Tony's apartment near the University of Wisconsin Milwaukee campus. We'd have a great time visiting, talking mostly about the book we were writing. Later, we'd walk to a nearby restaurant to dine outdoors if the weather was nice. Then, later in the evening, I drove my car and he drove his to my home in Oak Creek, about a half-hour away. I'd spend time with my two teens who had usually just come home from school sporting events or hanging with their friends. Andrew, my youngest, was often spending the night with his father on weekends that year.

While Tony slept downstairs in Jeanne's room, I had the master bedroom upstairs. Nothing inappropriate was ever going to happen in my house as long as I had children still at home. Tony and I would get up early the next morning, have breakfast, and then head to my office downstairs to begin work on the book.

Tony talked while I typed. Later, after he left, I'd re-work, rewrite, rewrite, rewrite. The next Friday and Saturday we'd repeat the same pattern. Dinner out on Friday night, then drive to my house where we worked most of Saturday morning on the book and sometimes late into the afternoon. He usually went back to his apartment Saturday after we finished working, primarily because I had things to do with my children, including church on Sundays.

During Tony's time in Milwaukee, the Federal Marshals were in charge of his relocation program. On the first day of every month, they met him at the lagoon in front of Lake Michigan in downtown Milwaukee and handed him an envelope with ten $100 bills in it, his stipend per the agreement they had with him as a member of the Federal witness protection program.

The Marshals also found Tony a job as a night supervisor in a huge food warehouse, a job Tony grew to hate. The stress of the job made him physically sick. His personality changed, and he even talked of walking out of the relocation witness program just to get away from the job.

I felt so bad for Tony that I broke an unspoken rule and wrote a letter to the FBI agent in charge of the Milwaukee division, pleading for them to help Tony find another job.

With no usable birth certificate or social security card, a felony on his record, and no proof that he was who he said he was because of so many name changes, Tony needed their help to get a job, but when they got him the food warehouse supervisor's position, they'd warned him that that was the last job they would help him get.

When I reread the letter I wrote to the FBI Agent in charge I'm astounded at the courage I had back in 1989. Who in their right mind would write such a letter? I'm sure there's a file on me in the FBI office in Milwaukee with a note saying I'm a crazy woman, a pest who got in the way of Tony and his attempt to relocate successfully in the witness protection program.

Here's the letter in its entirety, which obviously is entirely too long.

February 23, 1989

Agent in Charge

Federal Bureau of Investigation
517 E. Wisconsin Ave.
Milwaukee, WI 53203

Dear Sir:

I am writing to you regarding Tony _____. I called your office February 21st and asked to speak to you or the agent in charge of Tony's case. I was given the run around and then ignored. No one in your office had the decency to call me to find out what I wanted. Instead, your men barged into Tony's life (a life filled with trauma right now, I might add) and forced him out of your program, including all rights to future protection. My God, at the very least, what you have done is chop down the

*entire forest to save one tree. If you don't under-
stand the analogy, let me explain.*

*Yes, Tony violated your precious FBI ethics, or
whatever you want to call it, by telling me about
his former life, but for the past ten months Tony
and I have had a loving, caring relationship. I am
no dummy—and believe me, there would never
have been a relationship after our first date if Tony
hadn't told me the truth about himself. The days of
the good ole boys withdrawing into the parlor with
their fat cigars and brandy to discuss things while
the women sit in the sewing circle are over in case
you hadn't noticed.*

*In other words, a man and a woman share things—
everything, in fact. Without that, there can be no
trust. Without trust, there is no basis for a relationship or communication. You, above all, should
know that.*

*From the very beginning, Tony knew he could trust
me. I am, according to him, the most honest person he's ever met in his life. I am a hard-working,
single mother of four. I support my children, care
for them, love them, work two jobs, and take care
of the 6-bedroom home that I own—and I do it
well. I am law-abiding, God-fearing, and above
all, honest. I would never breach the sacred trust
between Tony and myself. That's why Tony knew
when he confided in me he would never have to
worry about me as a security risk. He never will.*

*But the thing that absolutely amazes me about you
and your department is the fact that when I called
Tuesday to ask for some help for Tony, knowing
that he was in serious distress, instead of talking to*

me or even having an agent, any agent, talk to me, you send your guns over to Tony immediately, read him the riot act, and cut him off from everything. How can you sleep at night, knowing that all you care about is POLICY? To hell with people and their problems, eh?

Tony's problems go something like this: the job you so generously helped him get is a nightmare. Since December 21, he has been forced to work longer and longer hours with more and more responsibility piled on him every day. At this point, he leaves for work around 3:30 p.m., prepares for his night shift, puts in 10 or 11 hours on the job (which officially starts at 5 p.m.), drives home sometimes around 3 a.m., parks his car a half-mile or so from his apartment because at that time of night there are no parking spaces on the east side, and finally gets to sleep sometimes after 5 a.m. He's back up around noon, and by the time he prepares his lunch or breakfast and fixes a decent meal to take to work with him, it's time to get dressed to go to work again. This man, who is most definitely a morning person having risen at 5 a.m. most of his life, has not seen the morning sun for over two months. Or any sun, for that matter. He hasn't had any exercise for two months. If you know anything about Tony at all, you know he's a power walker and a jogger and that daily exercise is very important to him.

He has not had any relaxation to speak of, especially now that he's also working his days off because of the food warehouse strike in Columbus. He's had to hire and fire many men since he began the job, which adds to the constant tension. The working conditions remind him of prison, and he should know, right? Cold, gray, concrete walls and floors, an extremely noisy environment, and Neanderthal types (all men), who can only grunt and spout off in four-letter words. The code among the men he must supervise seems to be that the less work they can do, the happier they are. As supervisor, Tony has to constantly bark at them, which adds even more tension to his job.

In recent weeks, Tony has become more and more depressed. He does not even have a doctor in Milwaukee (the one he had retired or moved or something), much less someone he can talk to about these things. If he did, he wouldn't have time to see anyone, anyway. This week, he even pushed me out of his life. The stress of trying to keep a relationship going got the best of him. Since I have been his best and only friend in Milwaukee, I'm sure it was a decision based on the unbearable stress he is facing. He has lost weight, is physically ill, and still drags himself in to work every day.

On Tuesday when I saw him for a few minutes, he even mentioned leaving Milwaukee. Knowing his past record of taking off when things got too much for him, I decided to ask your office to help him. All I wanted was for you to understand what was happening to Tony because of this job. I wanted you to reconsider and perhaps help him find a day job that would allow him to at least have a life other than those dark warehouse walls. I honestly thought he was on the verge of a nervous breakdown. I know enough about the way the human mind functions to know that a human being cannot work that much with no time for exercise, recreation, or even the slightest bit of relaxation without catastrophic results. At the pace he is going, Tony will end up in a mental ward somewhere or do something foolish like returning to his old New York neighborhood to be with his family.

So, can you at least understand my concern? Can you understand that I felt my only alternative was to come to you and ask for your help? Instead of listening to me, you crash down on him even more, driving him further and deeper into depression. What you did is unforgivable. Hasn't he done enough for the government over the past 25 years? Because of his FBI involvement, he certainly has never been allowed to lead a normal life with a normal career. So, here he is, at age 50, starting at the bottom. An intelligent, organized man with definite leadership qualities in his first real job. His first chance at starting a real life. Because his only crime now is trusting me, you jerk away the only security he had left in this world.

I plead with you. Swallow your pride. In grade school, we all learned that there's an exception to every rule. The fact that Tony trusts me with his life's story should be the exception to your rule. He's entitled to that much, and so am I.

You might be interested to know that I am writing a book about Tony's life, fictionalized, of course. If you cut him off cold and refuse to protect him in the future, I'm sure he'll leave Milwaukee for good. When that happens, my book will change. Instead of Tony's life fictionalized, it will be the story of my life with Tony these past ten months. You can be sure it won't be fiction. You can also be sure that this letter will be included verbatim, as well as all the FBI antics that have involved Tony's life, and therefore my life, since April 16, 1988. A fascinating story, I can assure you.

I appeal to your sense of decency. Give Tony the protection he deserves and needs, especially when he has to go back to New York to see his family in the future. You have to admit that he has been a model relocated witness since coming to Milwaukee last February. I know I have been a good, stabilizing influence on him.

Also, please help him get another job. Now that you've cut him off the program, he feels forced to stay in this job that is physically, mentally, and emotionally a nightmare. If something doesn't change for him soon, I know he will either leave the state or suffer a serious breakdown.

Surely our noble Department of Justice cares more about people than policy. Please help Tony.

Sincerely,
Patricia Lorenz

Of course, I never heard a word from the FBI after I sent this letter. I'm sure whoever read it got a good laugh. I mean, really, my ridiculous letter was over 1500 words long. Maybe they didn't even bother to read it.

After that I called the Federal Marshal's office to ask them to help Tony, but the minute I told them his real name, they denied knowing him and hung up the phone. Minutes later, they called Tony and told him his security had been breached and that he had to leave Milwaukee immediately. They were definitely not happy that he'd told me his real name, considering the fact that the East Coast mob still had a $100,000 bounty on his life. The mob in those days didn't mess around when someone turned state's witness against them.

At any rate, a squad of Federal Marshals arrived at Tony's apartment within the hour, helped him pack, and drove him out of Milwaukee and out of my life.

He called me eight hours later from Peoria, Illinois, telling me what happened. I was devastated and quite angry at both the Federal Marshals and the FBI. Tony was eventually relocated to Tulsa, Oklahoma, where he enrolled in a one-year Licensed Practical Nurse program. He wrote to me often during that year—long, somewhat boring letters written on yellow legal tablets, complaining mostly about how difficult nursing school was.

More than a year later after he graduated, Tony appeared in my driveway, still driving the same old blue Toyota the Federal Marshals had purchased for him a few years earlier when he arrived in Milwaukee for the first time. I was in the front yard raking leaves with my new boyfriend Marty.

Tony gave me a big hug and seemed genuinely glad to see me. Even though he knew I was dating Marty he still asked if he could stay at my house for a couple weeks while he looked for a job. My three older children were all off to college in other states and towns so I had three empty bedrooms. I put Tony downstairs in my oldest daughter's room. He was the perfect gentleman. Each morning he got up, put on a suit and tie, and went looking for a job. He found one at a big nursing home and a few days later found an apartment in a neighborhood five miles from my house. I helped him move in, gave him a good-bye hug, and walked down the steps. That was the last time I ever saw Tony.

I heard a few years later that he'd dated an acquaintance of mine for a few months, then later heard that he'd been fired from the nursing home and moved on. I still wonder what happened to Tony, his career, and whether or not he's still in the relocation program. It might be fun to finish the book we started about his life. At the very least, he was the most interesting, most lively character of all the men I ever dated, and he certainly opened my eyes to a whole different world of characters, who grew up in Brooklyn wishing they could be real members of the mafia.

Perhaps the takeaway message here is this: if you're thinking about dating an ex-Mafioso wannabe or a man with any relationship whatsoever with a gang or, heaven forbid, the Mafia, don't do it. Unless, of course, you just want to have an interesting time for a while and not let it get too serious. As long as he treats you with kindness and respect and doesn't have too many problems of his own that you have to deal with, you might just consider it a blip in your journey to find the real man you want to spend the rest of your life with. After all, life is about choices. As long as you're both enjoying your time together and he doesn't break your heart, what's the harm? The year I spent as Tony's friend will always be up there among the strangest, most interesting, and most fun times of my life. Sometimes, it's okay to grab for a little gusto outside your comfort zone and step into a world you know nothing about.

Patricia Lorenz

.

Marty: Mr. Nice Guy

This chapter about Marty will be short, mainly because although he was a very nice man, he didn't challenge me intellectually. Even though we dated for 2 1/2 years I really don't remember any life-changing events or conversations that we had together. Perhaps the excitement that Tony brought to my life kept me from giving Marty a fair chance, but I just couldn't picture myself with Marty for the long haul.

I met Marty when a friend of mine, 80-something-year-old Barbara, begged me to go to her daughter's high school reunion with her daughter Susan. Susan wanted to go, but since she lived out of state and hadn't kept in contact with anyone in her high school class, she didn't know anyone to ask so that she wouldn't have to walk in alone. I didn't even know Barbara's daughter and felt very squeamish about attending a reunion like that with another woman for fear everyone there would think we were a lesbian couple. Remember, this was in the early 90's. Things were different then. Since I was in the midst of looking for Mr. Right, I wanted to keep my heterosexual options open. In the end, though, I simply didn't have the heart to turn down the simple request from my dear friend Barbara. So, I went.

Sitting next to me at the round dinner table was Marty, seven years my senior. His date, a member of the reunion class, was a platonic friend. He was also doing a favor by accompanying her to the event.

Marty and I started talking, and we soon realized that we lived less than a mile from each other. When he told me he had a boat and a bicycle, I became even more interested in finding out more about him.

We agreed to meet for a bike ride the next week, in August of 1991. We had a great ride in a lovely hilly park along the shore of Lake Michigan. We spent the rest of the summer biking and boating. Those carefree days in Marty's boat made it seem that life with him might not be so bad after all. However, when winter came and the outdoor fun ended, I began to notice that there wasn't enough in our relationship to keep me interested. He was a retired electric company employee, a widower with two of his 20-something adult daughters still living with him.

Marty genuinely liked my only child still at home, Andrew, who was eleven at the time. That certainly gave Marty few points in my book. Andrew's father had died in 1989, and I was happy to provide a good, kind father-type role-model for Andrew.

For the next 2 ½ years, I dated Marty and even took a 27-day car trip across America with him and Andrew. We drove to California to visit my oldest daughter and truly had the time of our lives sharing the driving and oohing and aahhing at the magnificent scenery between Wisconsin and California and back.

During those 2 1/2 years, Marty and I (and most often Andrew as well) attended college football games at the University of Wisconsin where my son Michael was in the marching band. We made a few trips to visit my daughter, who was a student at the University of Wisconsin in Stephens Point, but other than that, there wasn't a whole lot of adventure or intrigue about this man.

I had no intention of ever marrying Marty. When we did talk about it a couple times, I quickly changed the subject. I finally decided the only way we would ever really break up would be if I could find him a different woman. My friend Gail suggested one of her best friends, a nurse who had been divorced for many years. I introduced Marty to the woman. They hit it off, eventually got married, and, as far as I know are living happily ever after. I haven't seen Marty since the end of 1993.

See, I said this chapter would be short. I honestly can't remember one thing about our time together worthy of another paragraph. Don't get me wrong. Marty was a very, very nice man—kind, considerate, and thoughtful—but sometimes that's just not enough. If you find someone good, honest, and kindhearted and you are still not that interested, perhaps it is simply not the right time for you to get serious about a relationship. In my case, I knew that raising Andrew was my number one priority. Finding a husband for myself was definitely on the back burner during those years. I'm happy it worked out that way, believe me. Timing is everything.

Patricia Lorenz

7

The Personals

I not only answered dozens of ads in the newspaper personals section during the early to late 90's I also probably had 20 or more first dates with men. Safe, boring, one-time-only dates. Dates with men I never wanted to see again. Meeting men in the personals became more of a hobby than a serious way to find Mr. Right. Years later when newspaper personals gave way to on-line dating, I have to say the on-line ads worked a lot better. Getting to know someone via e-mails is easier than only getting to talk to them on the phone before you actually met face to face on a real date. On-line photos and in-depth writing conversations back and forth help you weed out the frogs.

One year during the 90's, a friend of mine and I even offered a writing class at a big writers' conference on how to write sizzling ads for the personals. I can't remember how many people showed up or what exactly we taught them, but here's our promo ad for the class.

Patricia Lorenz

======================================

HOW TO WRITE GREAT ADS FOR THE PERSONALS
SATURDAY, FEBRUARY 1ST FROM 1-3:30
If you've never written an ad for the Personals but you're
DESPERATELY SEEKING SOMEONE
this rib-splitting workshop is for you.
If you've been writing ads for years and keep meeting frogs
instead of a prince or a princess, this hands-on workshop will
help you get that dance card filled.
Two single women, both full-time professional writers,
who have had lots of fun with the personals for years,
will take you step-by-step toward landing
the date of your dreams.
You'll not only write a great ad during this class,
but we guarantee a laugh a minute and free refreshments.
You'll also get help with voice mail ads.
P.S. If you meet Mr. Right, you have to invite us to the wedding.

======================================

Once the 21st century rolled around and on-line dating became big business with match-making companies bragging about how many marriages they'd created, dating took on a life of its own. Seven years earlier, in 1993, Dr. John Gray published the self-help book, *Men Are from Mars, Women Are from Venus.* That book revolutionized the way we thought about how men and women interact and helped pave the way for more successful dating. After all, if we were going to start dating in midlife and beyond, we at least had to have a better knowledge of what makes men tick.

Dr. Gray explained that one of the biggest differences between men and women is how they cope with stress. Men become increasingly focused and withdrawn when they're experiencing stress. Women become increasingly overwhelmed and emotional. Men feel better by solving problems. Women feel better by talking about problems.

The book goes on to explain that when a woman becomes upset or is stressed by her day, to find relief she seeks someone she trusts and then talks in great detail about everything that went wrong that day. When she shares feelings of being overwhelmed, she suddenly feels better. A woman is not ashamed of having problems. A woman's ego is not dependent on looking competent but rather on being in loving relationships. We women openly share feelings of being overwhelmed, confused, hopeless, and exhausted. Men do not. A woman feels good about herself when she has loving friends with whom to share her feelings and problems, but a man feels good when he can solve his problems on his own in his cave.

When a woman talks to a man about problems, the man assumes she is holding him responsible. The more problems, the more he feels blamed. He doesn't realize she's talking to feel better and that he doesn't have to do a thing but sit there and nod his head supportively.

Dr. Gray explains that men talk about problems for only two reasons: they are blaming someone or they are seeking advice. If a woman is really upset, the man assumes she is blaming him. He draws his sword to protect himself from the attack. If she seems less upset, he assumes she is asking for advice. He becomes Mr. Fix-It and tries to solve her problems. The real problem, however, is that we women don't want the men in our lives solving our problems. We just want to talk about them. We aren't blaming them or seeking advice. We just need to talk it out.

When you're carving out a relationship with a man, whether it's someone you just met on-line or someone you've been dating for years, it's important to know some of the basic differences in the two genders.

For the most part women **talk to think**. I know firsthand that I can be in a room full of people who are having an interesting discussion about this or that. I'll find myself joining the conversation, and sometimes just by talking I can change my opinion 180 degrees. I'm like most women. We think as we talk, and we find it easy to rearrange our opinions while we're talking.

Men, on the other hand, **think to talk**. Usually they don't say a thing until they've thought about the issue long enough to form an educated opinion. Only then are they able to verbally express themselves. When they do talk, it is to convey or gather information. They must think first and talk later.

Did you ever notice that a man will generally stop talking when he's upset? He needs to retreat to his cave to cool off and ponder his thoughts. Once he's thought things through, he'll come back to you with some well-thought-out opinions on the matter at hand.

I read somewhere years ago that men, on average, say 7,000 words a day. Women say 20,000 words a day. The thing is, men do not want to listen to—and probably can't even process—our 20,000 words. That's why we women must find, nourish, and enjoy friendships with other women. We can talk to our hearts' content, change our opinions willy-nilly while we're talking, and solve almost every problem in any relationship we ever have with our women friends.

So, if you're out there experiencing on-line dating or just being set up with a few good men by your women friends, make sure you're also taking the time to nourish friendships with many women. Close friendships with other women provide the gold threads that help you create the fabric of an amazing relationship with a man. We women need close friendships with other women in order to survive this world of dating. Believe me, your women friends will be the ones who will help you create a relationship with a man that sizzles.

Patricia Lorenz

The Crash Pad

When the phone rang that day in March of 1994, I had no idea that my life was about to change and that more men than I could possibly imagine would enter my life. It was my friend and neighbor, Bruce Swezey, a part-time pilot for the Air National Guard who had just been hired as a full-time pilot for Milwaukee's Midwest Express Airlines.

"So, Bruce, how's ground school going?"

"That's why I'm calling, Pat. It's terrific, but I have a favor to ask. There are 12 guys in my class from all over the country. Most of them are living in flea-bag hotels to save money while they're in ground school. You've got extra bedrooms now that your older kids are on their own. Why don't you open up a *crash pad* for a couple of the guys during our ground school, just for a month or so?"

I gasped when he suggested it. "Houseguests for that long? Would I have to cook for them?" Quite frankly, Bruce's idea didn't sound like much fun.

"No. Tracy and I put two guys in our extra room in the basement. They eat out mostly. We don't even see them unless we get together to study. They're great guys, Pat.

One just retired from the Air Force. Another was a Navy pilot. They're married and have kids, and I know they'd be happier in a home environment instead of those seedy motels they're in."

"Well, let me think about it. I'll talk to Andrew."

"No problem, Pat. Call me when you decide."

It was true, Andrew, who was 14 at the time, and I were banging around in our six-bedroom house. Andrew's father died when Andrew was just nine years old, and as the three older kids left for college, we went from a family of six to a family of two in just a few years. I used one bedroom for my writing room office, but three bedrooms and a full bath downstairs weren't even being used.

Over the years I'd worried about how a single-parent mom could possibly teach her son how to be a man. My dad, brother, brother-in-law, and uncles all lived out of state, and we didn't see them often enough for them to have much impact on Andrew. Even Andrew's older brother, Michael, eight years his senior, was busy finishing his last two years at the University of Wisconsin two hours away. With Michael's two part-time jobs and his full-time class schedule, he rarely made it home except for holidays. Without a doubt, Andrew could use a few regular male role models in his life.

But I still wasn't sure about the idea of having two or three men move in downstairs. How would I feel about my loss of privacy? Would they interrupt me in my home office? Who would clean their bathroom and bedrooms? Not me.

I finally sat down and typed up a list of *Crash Pad Do's and Don'ts*. I figured that even if they were only going to be living in my home for a month or so, I'd better make it clear from the beginning what I expected of them and what they could expect of me. On that list, I said they'd have to do their own cooking, but they could use my pots, pans, dishes, spices, condiments, and milk. I didn't want 3-gallon jugs of milk cluttering up my refrigerator. I'd provide and wash sheets and towels for them, but they'd have to remake their own beds, clean the downstairs bathroom and vacuum, and dust their bedrooms.

I talked to Andrew again, who needed to be reassured that he'd still be able to watch TV downstairs in the family room even if the pilots were here.

"What if I want to have my friends over, Mom?"

"No problem. The pilots have to study every night, son. They're in ground school, remember? They'll probably be out studying with friends or in the quiet of their bedrooms. If they want to come out and watch TV with you while your friends are here, what difference does it make?"

I was starting to like the idea that for the first time in years Andrew would have to learn how to share our big house with others. For the past few years, he'd had the run of the place and had not learned the art of being considerate of others' needs in a home. I had a feeling the next month would be good for Andrew.

I called Bruce. "Okay, my friend, we'll do it. Send the two most stellar pilots over to check us out. If they like the place, they can stay here. I figure I can survive anything for 30 days."

The next day Wade and Ron moved in. A week later, Lyle joined them. The Lorenz Crash Pad was in full swing.

Wade was a retired Air Force pilot whose family lived in Colorado Springs. He'd been one of General Norman Schwarzkopf's personal pilots during Desert Storm so I knew I didn't have to bother checking his credentials. Wade had interesting stories to share with Andrew and me during those early evenings when we were all cooking, gabbing, and laughing in the kitchen while we fixed our individual dinners.

Wade had also been an instructor at the Air Force Academy, a place we'd visited the summer before and where Andrew was dreaming of going to college. He and Wade had lots of academy conversations during those meal preparations. Wade was a good-looking, soft-spoken man with a small frame. Truth be told, all of the pilots who stayed at my crash pad were good looking. There were times during those years that I wondered if it were an airline hiring requirement that they be good-looking and well-built. Or was it because I was a single woman, and to me those men in my home were such a breath of fresh air that they all just seemed to be good-looking to me.

Ron was a Navy pilot whose family lived in Dallas. He'd flown Top Gun type planes as well as helicopters during his career and was also a well of information as Andrew pumped him with questions about military life. Ron gave Andrew a play-by-play account of what it was like to land a helicopter on an aircraft carrier in the middle of the ocean.

Ron was married to a stunning Jamaican woman and had two teenage boys and a younger daughter. Once when I was on vacation, Ron brought his two teenage sons to stay with him in my home for a week while he was on reserve. He was in the process of moving his family to Milwaukee from Texas, and his wife had gotten their house all ready to show for the Realtor. She didn't want the boys messing it up so she sent them up to my house. I was teaching at a writer's conference in Missouri that week so Ron figured having his boys there wouldn't bother me. He also didn't bother to ask my permission to bring the boys.

Trouble is, it was the hottest week of the summer. I returned home to find rings from wet glasses all over my wooden furniture and a glass of moldy milk in the corner of the family room. The tape recorders in my office closet had been taken out and used by the boys. They also broke the neighbor's basketball backboard. I was furious and told Ron I was running a crash pad for pilots, not for teenage boys, and that they would have to leave. He finally sent them back home, and a few weeks later he moved into a house in a Milwaukee suburb with his family.

I ran into Ron a few years later on a flight from Phoenix to Milwaukee where he was the captain flying the plane. He gave me a big hug and showed me photos of his kids. The oldest had just graduated from the U. S. Naval Academy.

Lyle was a 40-something, blond, medium-built pilot who did not have a college education—very unusual for a commercial pilot. He had worked his way to the top plane ratings one small step at a time, working for a number of small carriers. Once, when working for a tiny local carrier, he also had a part-time job delivering suitcases from the airport for a taxi company. Lyle was very methodical, extremely knowledgeable about the airplane systems, and fastidious almost to the point of being nerdy. He studied new material like a crazy man whenever it was issued by the company. The joke around the airline during those years was that if anyone had a question about any system or maintenance problem the answer was, "Ask Lyle."

Eventually Lyle moved to a small apartment in South Milwaukee so he could have peace and quiet to study intently for his coming upgrade to Captain. Lyle was a very frugal soul who never turned down a free meal, free beer, or anything I had to offer in the way of eats. He was also very helpful in getting me friend passes although he made sure I paid him to the penny what he had to pay on his taxes, state and federal as well as social security, for each standby pass ticket.

When Lyle, a vegetarian who hadn't done much cooking for himself moved in, we all teased him about the way he made spaghetti. He threw pasta into cold water and boiled it to smithereens. Then, he poured refrigerator-cold spaghetti sauce directly onto the drained pasta and started eating. Wade, who was a good cook, gave Lyle a few tips about boiling the water first and heating the sauce before putting it on the pasta. Andrew watched the whole process and saw firsthand that it's okay for real men to cook and that it's okay to make mistakes along the way. During those dinner preparations, I could almost see Andrew's sense of humor blossoming before my eyes as he watched and chatted with those macho professional men kibitzing in our kitchen.

When Ron and Wade left for a couple of weeks of simulator training in another city after their ground school, they both asked if they could come back and stay at our house until the end of the summer when they could get their families moved to Milwaukee. I said "Yes, of course!"

By now we'd become great friends and there seemed to be no reason not to continue the arrangement. Besides, Andrew and I were planning some trips that summer, and I felt good knowing these guys would keep an eye on things for me while were gone.

Over Mother's Day weekend, Wade's wife came to visit her husband, and, of course, I invited her to stay at the house with all of us. She and I became such great friends that I asked her if she'd like to come back and stay for a week in June so she could play mother hen to Andrew while I taught at a writer's conference out of state. She loved the idea of spending a whole week with her hubby and even brought her daughter who was a year younger than Andrew. The two adults and two teens had a blast while I was gone, and I was able to relax completely, knowing that my son was in very capable, loving hands.

As the summer progressed, Rusty moved in to join Wade, Ron and Lyle. The five of us enjoyed one humorous conversation after another on a daily basis. Andrew saw firsthand just how easy it is for men and women to be good platonic friends.

When Rusty still owned his own parachute jumping school, he had made hundreds upon hundreds of jumps, which was very impressive to my son Andrew. Like all the pilots who stayed at the Lorenz Crash Pad, Rusty was a very interesting, fun, and intelligent man. He was at our home for six months while he was on reserve right after getting hired at Midwest Express Airlines. Then, he moved his family to the Milwaukee area from Kansas City. His wife Heather was an attorney who had both of their daughters in her early 40's, then quit work to stay home and mother full-time. Rusty and Heather remained friends of ours for many years until I lost track of them after I moved to Florida.

When Wade and Ron moved their families to Milwaukee at the end of the summer, they spread the word about the Lorenz Crash Pad to other pilots, who asked if they could stay with us. Before long, we had six: Lyle, Bob, Dave, Eric, Rob, and Patrick. Dave eventually got a job with UPS and moved back to his home in Philadelphia. Patrick had a few mishaps and lost his job with the company and moved back to Florida. As soon as one pilot would leave, another on my waiting list would ask to join the crew at our house.

When Bob was using our home as his crash pad during the early years when Andrew was a youngster, Andrew and he worked on plans for a treehouse and put the thing together one week when Bob was on reserve. Another time, he was on reserve for six months, during which time he enjoyed golfing, fishing, and shopping for computers. He complained about not being home with his family, but I know he was enjoying that golf. He also helped me decide which computer to buy for my writing business.

Once, when I was having a party that night, I walked downstairs to discover Bob vacuuming the family room. "'Hey Bob," I said, "You don't have to do that."

He replied, "I was bored; besides, I know you're having that party tonight and just thought I'd help a little."

Be still my heart. He made me promise not to tell his wife, Mary, that he was being so helpful. "Wouldn't want to ruin my image," he laughed. I was secretly glad that Andrew saw firsthand that *real* men do housework.

Bob lived with his wife and two sons in northern Wisconsin in a beautiful home on a lake. He used my crash pad for about three years. At that point, he was able to bid a schedule that only had him overnighting in Milwaukee one or two nights a month so he decided to stay in an inexpensive motel across from the airport.

By 1997, I had seven pilots and a navigator: Doug from Michigan, Rob from Vermont, Troy from Omaha, Jim from Texas, Rodney from Kansas City, Matt from Florida, Eric from Michigan, and Theresa, a navigator for the Air National Guard.

Theresa was a former math teacher who spent a number of evenings at our house, helping my son with algebra and geometry. As a devout Christian, she also drew us into interesting conversations about faith, religion, and the right way to live in today's world. When Theresa left the house in her green Air Force jumpsuit to go to her navigator's job in a KC-135 refueling plane, I was glad that Andrew saw that women can have important macho jobs and still be successful, happy wives and mothers. I was also thankful for the spiritual role modeling Theresa provided for my son.

From 1994-2004, over 40 pilots stayed at our house in Milwaukee. When Andrew left for college in Arizona in 1998, I treasured the pilots even more. With an empty nest, I was able to travel more, and the pilots were all very generous with their standby passes so I could fly for pennies on the dollar from coast to coast to visit all four of my children.

The pilots helped make my empty nest house much livelier. In addition to the fun they brought into my life, I never had to worry about my house, mail, or yard when I left town for a weekend or weeks at a time. The pilots kept an eye on everything.

Once when I was away for a week, the downstairs flooded when the pilot's shower backed up. Jim and Dave ran the shop-vac off and on all morning to help get the water out. Jim also split wood for the wood-burner, took phone messages for me, and shared his vittles whenever he cooked a big meal.

When Lyle stayed with us, he would talk to Andrew about cars and how they work. Since I don't know a dip stick from a hockey stick, the conversations alone were eye-openers to my son. Sometimes, Lyle even asked Andrew to help when he did minor maintenance on his car.

Dave, a Polish Catholic Democrat who lived in Philadelphia with his wife Barb, had a great sense of humor. Andrew often heard Dave and me yucking it up about the latest boondoggle in the world of politics or discussing our common religious backgrounds. He was a real rabble-rouser when it came to wanting a pilot's union at Midwest. When Andrew joined the young Republicans club at school, Dave never let up, teasing him mercilessly about his political mistake. Andrew loved it and learned to kibitz with the best of 'em.

Once, when I had to be out of town one weekend and left Andrew in the hands of the pilots, I reminded Dave that Andrew's only rule was that he couldn't have any friends in the house while I was gone. Dave grinned and said, "Okay, no problem. Andrew, you gotta keep the party at least 50 feet from the front door."

We all laughed. I was secretly glad that there would be one or two pilots around all weekend, responsible guys Andrew could gab with, watch movies and cook with while I was gone.

Doug talked to Andrew about finances. "Andrew, you should definitely start investing your money in mutual funds as soon as you get out of college." I'm not sure how much of Doug's financial management lectures sunk into Andrew's 16-year-old head, but at least my son was learning that men have all sorts of interests and ways of doing things and that financial planning is an important part of life.

Matt, who was born in Germany, had a distinctive German accent. He lived in my home full time for a couple months in 1994 and then bought a house in a neighboring town. A few years later, he moved to Florida and came back to my crash pad to stay.

Matt used very strong shaving lotion, and I could tell whenever the front door opened that it was Matt coming in. He was a tall guy with a pretty good sense of humor. A political soul who was looking forward to having a pilot's union, he enjoyed rapping about problems within the company with the other pilots.

Eric, who lived in Michigan, had an easy-going personality and a great sense of humor. Andrew and I both enjoyed spending an evening with him in the family room, watching a movie and eating pizza. Eric's wife stayed at our house a few times when they were flying out of Milwaukee on vacation. Once when Andrew and I were in Michigan, Eric and Cathy invited us to spend the night in their beautiful home. We did, and the friendship between our two families solidified.

Eric stayed at our home for over four years but wasn't really considered one of the regular crash padders because as a Captain high on the seniority list he got such good trips that he rarely had to be in Milwaukee overnight, maybe once every two months at most. Eric liked to drink and usually popped a beer or two or three the minute he arrived after a long day's work. He was very careful, however, never to drink within the 10-hour limit before a flight, regulated by the Federal Aviation Administration.

He was an easy-going, very friendly guy who, because he only saw me every couple of months, gave me a big hug every time he walked in the door. Unfortunately, Eric's career as a pilot ended when he died suddenly of a heart attack on the golf course at age 53.

Jim, a former Wisconsinite who now lives in Texas with his wife, was (and no doubt still is) a big Dallas Cowboys fan. Of course, I'm a dyed-in-green-wool fan of America's Team, the Green Bay Packers. Every weekend during football season, Jim drew goofy pictures of the Cowboys and Packers on the white board next to our front door. The Cowboys had their worst season in six years in 1997, which meant I was in my heyday. I found a large, full-color photo on a calendar of an old rickety outhouse out in the woods where somebody had painted COWBOYS on the front door. I made a sign that said, "Future Headquarters of the Dallas Cowboys," taped it to the top of the outhouse picture, and put it up on the wall just inside my front door. Jim took it all in stride. Football season was never more fun than it was that year, the year the Packers won the Super Bowl.

When Steve, Dave, Dale, and George were all staying at the crash pad, we discovered a mutual love of Asian food. Steve, whose last name is Hong, was born in South Korea and could make Korean food like a pro. On the nights when our begging resulted in Steve's filling the house with the aroma of kimchi or a rich beef stew called kari-kari served with rice and hot pepper sauce, we all gathered at the dining room table hungry enough to eat Milwaukee.

When Steve took a job with another airline and moved back to the East Coast, George, Dave, and I would visit our favorite Thai restaurant and talk about the good old days when Steve introduced us to the wonders of Korean cooking.

The Lorenz Crash Pad lasted ten full years. Running that crash pad for the pilots was a little bit of heaven for a single woman like me. Sometimes, it felt like having lots of younger brothers hanging around my house off and on each month. Other times, I basked in the joy of having men closer to my own age filling my family room with lively, intelligent conversation. They cared for me, helped me around the house, provided security, and helped pay my house taxes and utilities with their donations to the crash pad fund during those ten years.

Fifteen or twenty nights a month when there would be one, two, three, or, once-in-a-great-while, four pilots staying at our home, it was alive with laughter, fun, conversation, and the best role models I could have asked for my son before he left for college. Without a doubt, the crash pad experience opened up our lives to new experiences, attitudes, and wonderful warm friendships. Because of those charming men who came in and out of my home, I rarely dated during those ten years. I cherished the respect and kindness I received from all those pilots and quite frankly didn't feel the need to delve into the personals to surround myself with men I could date. More than at any other time in my life, having men in my home, men I could trust 100%, who were definitely not hitting on me, helped me learn to simply enjoy men.

My rule for inviting pilots into my crash pad was that they had to be happily married with kids at home. I didn't want any funny business going on and definitely did not want pilots bringing women they might be dating into my home. I also wanted men who would be great role models for my teenage son.

For ten years, the men in my life were true friends, none of whom were available as dating partners but who taught me what real men are like. It was positively delightful having fun with lots of different men with absolutely no sexual tension involved.

There's a verse in *Hebrews* that puts it all into perspective. It says, "Don't forget to be kind to strangers, for some who have done this have entertained angels without realizing it!" (*Hebrews* 13:2, *The Living Bible*.)

I'll tell you one thing. The Lorenz Crash Pad was definitely a place where the angels I entertained provided me with a lot more than I provided for them. I guess that's just how it works when you step out in faith and open up your home and your heart to strangers, especially strangers who are pilots.

Patricia Lorenz

Six Years of Jack

Jack and I met at the condo pool in Largo, Florida in April 2003 while I was vacationing there, staying in the condo I co-owned with my brother and sister. I was still living in Milwaukee, Wisconsin, but ever since 2002 when we bought the Florida condo, I visited the land of sun, sand, sea, surf, and glorious sunsets 3-4 times a year, thanks to the friend passes from the pilots in my crash pad back home.

At the pool, Jack and I treaded water in the deep end while we talked about our children: my four and his six. We bragged about our grandchildren. We talked about the church we both belonged to where he was the head usher. We discussed the fact that we both liked to travel. He shared stories about the many cruises he and his wife Jane had taken over the years.

I only got to meet Jane one time at the pool. Unfortunately she had been diagnosed with liver disease. A year later, April 2004, she died peacefully in the hospital. Back home in Milwaukee, I sent Jack a sympathy card with just a few paltry words scrawled at the bottom. How could I, who had been married, divorced and annulled twice, and never lived with either husband longer than seven years even begin to understand the pain of losing a spouse you loved with all your heart for 43 years? I couldn't come close to touching what must have been unbearable sadness. After all, it had been the longevity and joyfulness of his marriage that fascinated me about Jack in the first place.

The next time I visited Florida, a month after Jane's death, I saw Jack sitting alone at the pool in a lounge chair. I walked over to offer my condolences. He hugged me and said, "Thank you so much for your kind words on the card."

I wanted to know more about Jane: her life, her illness, and her death. How were their children coping? What about their youngest daughter, pregnant with her second child? How was she doing?

I kept asking questions. Jack kept talking. Before long, I understood that he probably needed someone outside the family to talk to, and so, with the help of my many questions, Jack talked to me that day at the pool for five straight hours.

The next day he was there, in the same spot when I arrived at the pool for my daily swim. He talked. I listened. He cried. I nodded my head and tried to understand his pain. Then, I shared a little of my own life and background, especially about how hard it was when my second husband, the father of my fourth child, died when Andrew was only nine years old. We had things in common, Jack and I, and we talked again without stopping for five hours.

The third day when I arrived at the pool, he motioned me over the minute I walked inside the fence. "Here, I brought you a cold soda," he proclaimed as the opener for that day's four-hour conversation.

On the fourth day, Jack and I were in the deep end of the pool, hanging onto the ledge with our elbows, talking more about the fragility of life and the importance of going on. Suddenly, this man who had opened so much of his heart and soul to me over the past four days asked me if he could ask me a question.

"Of course," I said, curious as to why he needed permission to ask me a question.

He took a deep breath. "Would you ever be interested in pursuing a relationship with me?"

I couldn't speak. I'd been single since 1985 when Harold moved out. I'd raised four children as a single parent. In nineteen years, I'd only dated two men: Tony for eight months and Marty for 2½ years. After that, I hadn't had more than one date with any man for the past 12 years. A relationship was the furthest thing from my mind.

The only thing I could think to do at the moment was raise my arms up over my head, inhale as much air as I could into my lungs, and sink slowly to the bottom of the pool. That's exactly what I did.

Oh, my gosh! Oh, my gosh! This poor man! What am I going to say? What does he mean? Why is he asking this? He loved his wife so much, and she just died five weeks ago. How could he ask me such a thing? Why? What should I say to him? I had no idea how to respond.

At that second, I had to come up for air so I surfaced and gasped for breath. I looked at Jack and asked, "What exactly do you have in mind?"

"I have no idea. I just know that I like talking to you. I also know three things. One, I loved my wife very much. Two, she's gone, and she's never going to come back to me. Three, Jane would not want me to sit around feeling sorry for myself. She would want me to be happy. I'm a realist, that's all."

"But it's only been five weeks since she died. You can't possibly mean that you want to start dating this soon."

"No, I guess not. Besides, even if we did go out, we would have to be very discreet. My children are hurting, and they need more time to grieve. I did most of my grieving this past year before Jane died. There were months and months when we both knew it didn't look good. She knew how much I loved her and cared for her, but she was also the type to say, 'Get on with your life, Jack.'"

He continued slowly. "I'd just like to see you, that's all."

"Well, then, why don't we go for a bike ride?" I suggested, thinking that seemed like a safe alternative to dating. "We have four bikes in our condo shed. I'm sure we could find one that would work for you. Let's bike over to the Gulf and go for a swim."

"I haven't been on a bike in years, but it sounds like fun. How about if I make a couple bologna sandwiches? I have some really good German bologna and rye bread."

"That's fine, I'll make the drinks. I'd like mustard on both slices of bread. No mayonnaise," I prattled.

An hour later, Jack and I met again, gathered the bikes, placed our picnic in the bike basket, and took off on the 2-mile jaunt to the Gulf. When we sat down on the sand on our beach towels, I opened the sandwich. Mustard on both slices. I looked over at Jack and smiled. *Here's a man who really pays attention*, I thought to myself. If you want to know the truth, I started falling in love with him at that very moment.

We were together every day for the rest of my 3-week visit to Florida. No two people talked more than we did during those days. A month later, I returned to my favorite place on earth for another three weeks. Knowing that I'd been dreaming of living in Florida fulltime for years, Jack told me about a condo for sale in his building. I looked at it twice. My belief that one should follow your dreams while you're still awake and my disdain for those long, 6-month winters in Wisconsin were the catalysts for my making an offer on the condo. My 6-bedroom empty-nest house in Wisconsin sold in two weeks.

The next month, in August of 2004, Jack came to Wisconsin to help me get rid of most of my furnishings at my second huge rummage sale. Then, he helped me pack the rest. We arrived in Florida 30 hours before Hurricane Frances. The next week, it was Hurricane Ivan and the next week, Hurricane Jeanne. I loved the wind, rain, and excitement of each storm, mainly because none of them sliced through my new neighborhood with a direct hit.

What was a direct hit, however, was my relationship with Jack. We had our ups and downs during the next few years, but I'm just glad that this man had the courage to ask me the question that caused me to sink to the bottom of the deep end of the pool for a minute while I pondered the rest of my life.

I fell in love with Jack in 2004 when I was fifty-eight years old and he was sixty-seven. I learned that when it comes to love, it's never too late to fall for someone even if it's the second or third time around.

When I first met him at the pool before his wife died, I thought he was at least 15 years older than I was. That, plus the fact that he was happily married to a wonderful woman, kept me from even giving him a second look. After his wife died and he had made it obvious that he was interested in me, I finally asked him how old he was. Nine years older. Since my first husband was seven years older and my second husband was seventeen years older I figured perhaps something in between might be OK.

Ladies, a word of advice: Once you hit 50, consider only dating men who are your age or a few years younger.

As the next few years passed of being Jack's neighbor in the same condo building, I have to say those nine years between us seemed to get in the way, at least in my mind. I'm a very active soul who works hard to stay healthy by eating right and exercising every day. Jack was a sedentary soul who seemed to be put on this earth to watch sports on TV from a recliner. So, that blissful phase of our lives didn't last. It never does, right? Every relationship has ups and downs. Within the year, I admit to making a list of reasons why I could never marry him. I've always been a list-maker. It helps me think through things.

In July 2010, because of my negativity about the relationship, six years after we started dating, Jack ended it. Slam! Bam!

Truth be told, Jack did not work up the courage to break up on his own. On a 5-day cruise with ten members of his family, two of his female relatives told Jack things I had supposedly said about his deceased wife. All of it was absolutely untrue and so out of line that to this day I am still dumbfounded and hurt. I had never once in all the years I'd known or dated Jack ever said or thought an unkind thing about his wonderful wife who was an amazing mother, grandmother, and friend to many. To do so would be unbelievably unkind, totally untrue, and something I would never consider doing. It also would have been relationship suicide. Jack used that short beach-side conversation with his relatives, however, as the catalyst to end our 6-year relationship. He had to save face with them. I also think that deep down in his soul he wondered who else was out there for him to date. After all, he'd had me in his back pocket since five weeks after his wife died.

Within days of our break-up, Jack was online looking for other women. In less than a month, he had another woman at his side, spending the weekends in his condo just 57 steps from my own. The pain of watching her enter his condo was almost more than I could bear. For eleven months, I stood at my dining room window and watched the comings and goings of the man I thought I had loved for six years. Those months were a blur of anguish brought on by self-flagellation because I'd stayed too long in the relationship. I have to admit, though, that the pain of seeing him every day and missing the good times was worse. Many days, I saw him numerous times. After all, we only lived 57 steps apart, and neither of us wanted to sell our condos and move from our beloved neighborhood.

Most mornings, we were both in the big pool together across the street, doing our usual water aerobics class. I was so hurt and angry by the break-up and his dating that I often didn't even say hello to him even if we were the only two who showed up for class. It's hard to describe the angst in my heart during those months.

I flip-flopped between being angry at myself for spending the previous six years with Jack and missing him more than I could even express to my friends and family. I wondered every day, *Had I settled for less than I wanted, needed, or was attracted to? But if that were true, why did I miss him so much?* I kept telling myself that I deserved someone who was my equal age-wise, someone who could keep up with me adventure-wise, and someone who had the same healthy lifestyle and the same interests, but then I'd look out my window, hoping I'd see him. I looked out that window so many times that eventually I knew I was still in love with the man. But he was gone, in another relationship with another woman.

Eventually, after a few long painful months I decided that since Jack was dating and even had the nerve to bring his new girlfriend to a few of our clubhouse events that I also attended, I should get my act together and also start dating.

So, like many people my age looking for a good partner in life, I went on-line to a free dating site. Oh, my!

10

The Journal

As a woman in my 60s who was now at the mercy of the Internet to help me find a nice man to date, I decided to keep a journal of the experience. It was actually a small notebook purchased to keep notes on the various men I met online, notes that would help me decide if I really wanted to meet the man in person after e-mailing and then talking to them on the phone.

My first entry in that journal says, "Jack and I were both guilty of letting a dead-end relationship linger long past its shelf life because the task of ending it was just too difficult." That must have been one of my hurt and angry days and not one of my looking-out-the-window-wishing-he-would-appear days.

I made a few philosophical observations in my journal, things like "We become attached to what's familiar and hold on to the safe and predictable even if it's bad for us." Looking back on that time in my life, I'd say those words are very accurate.

Patricia Lorenz

Word of advice: If you've settled for something that's safe and predictable but not necessarily happy, get out of there now. Life is short.

Page three of my journal reads, "I am free. Free to be who I am. No more agonizing. No more drama. No more walking on eggshells. No more regrets. No more time wasted on someone who doesn't appreciate me for who I really am. Freedom means I can now be myself. Freedom to follow my own dreams."

Page four reads, "Doubt means *don't* every time. I doubted this relationship would work so many times and for so many years. Why didn't I know that doubt means don't? Two great people can get together and have horrible chemistry."

Page five reads, "What about him is more valuable than making yourself feel whole again? Backsliding means you can have me with no strings attached. Honor. Dignity. Grace."

I suppose I was chastising myself for the times over the past six years that Jack and I had had disagreements, broken up for a few hours or maybe a day, and then rushed right back into each other's arms. I think all couples tend to thrive on a bit of chaos. After all, making up is so much fun, and in your 60s and 70s, it's comforting to be back with the one you think you love. Maybe that's true no matter what age you are.

On the next page in my dating journal, I listed seven commandments that I think I culled from a book for people who had just broken up

1. Don't see or talk to him for 60 days.
2. Get a break-up buddy.
3. Get rid of his stuff.
4. Get your ass in motion every day.

5. Don't take the break-up into the world.
6. No backsliding.
7. It won't work unless I am #1.

Well, I couldn't do number one because we lived just 57 steps apart. Quite often, I saw him coming and going from his condo or walking across the street to the pool. Of course, it was painful. A root canal would be less painful, but there wasn't a thing I could do about it.

I did get a break-up buddy, my friend Brenda. She's somebody I could rant and rave to and who wouldn't judge me for my craziness. It's important to have a friend like that, someone who loves you unconditionally, and who won't spread your angst to anyone else.

I'm telling you all this because you're obviously looking for a life partner, and, believe me, you will probably have to go through a lot of men like I did to find the one you want to wake up with every morning. Going through those experiences means a few break-ups along the way. So, pay attention.

Pondering commandment number three, *getting rid of his stuff*, did seem like a good idea. The less you have around you that reminds you of him (or her), the better. So, I took a bag of his stuff down to him, and he returned the favor with a whole garbage bag full of my stuff. The exchange was hurtful.

The rest of those seven steps are self-explanatory and good advice. They can be put into five simple words: *Get on with your life.* Needlepoint it if you have to, but get on with your life. Put it on the refrigerator, the bathroom mirror, and your front door: *Get on with your life.*

So, I did. I signed up for an on-line dating site, and let the fun begin.

The first guy I met was Greg. After a few somewhat interesting e-mails back and forth and two phone calls I agreed to meet him at Panera Bread. He bought me a green iced tea and kept jumping up from his seat to pick up more of the free samples of bread to eat. Then, he divulged that he eats most of his meals at Burger King, lives in a single-wide trailer, does no exercise, doesn't travel, and sells insurance. That might have been the fastest date in the history of the world. There wasn't one thing about him, including his looks, that I liked.

Message to you: If there is absolutely no chemistry when you meet someone, don't waste your time or theirs. Get out of there as fast as you can.

The next man I met, Ned, deserves his own chapter. So, here it is.

11

Ned

Ned sent me an e-mail telling me he liked my on-line profile and thought we had a lot in common. He wanted to meet, talk, visit and get to know each other better. I responded that I was busy that week but would be willing to have a short meet-and-greet the following week.

Ned wrote, "Thanks for your email. I understand your schedule. No problem, and next week meeting would be great. We can get in contact Sunday or Monday and decide plans. Have a great day!!"

I wrote: "Sounds good. Question: Is that your big dog in your line of pictures on the dating site? I don't have any pets (not allowed in my building), and I've never owned a dog. I love animals in the wild but not particularly in the home. Have a great weekend. I'll wait to hear from you Sunday or Monday."

Ned responded, "My dog's name is Barney. I will email you Sunday or Monday, but can we plan on Tuesday or Wednesday to meet?"

We met the following week for lunch at a nearby restaurant. Ned was short. He said he was 5'9" but was actually more like 5'7". Like many men who have reached or passed middle age, he was balding with a chunky round face, rosy cheeks, and a bit of a round body. He may not have been my ideal man in the looks department, but I certainly did enjoy talking to him. He'd had many interesting experiences as a boat captain, traveled around the world, had an iffy relationship with his daughters, and seemed to be in the middle of finding his next job. His previous jobs had been a bit marginal. I eventually got the impression that there might have been some funny business going on with some wheeler dealers overseas as a sidebar to his job of selling boat insurance. However, he was interesting enough and smart enough about world events that I wanted to keep seeing him. At that point in my life, I needed someone to entertain my brain with stimulating conversation.

After our meeting, Ned wrote: "So nice to hear from you. I also really enjoyed our meeting and talk. I probably talked too much but enjoyed your stories very much. It is interesting to note the commonality of our past as well as our love for the water. I look forward to our next meeting and in the meantime wish you the best in your travels and a safe return. Take care, Ned."

I replied, "Enjoyed meeting you and, as a sea lover myself, especially enjoyed hearing your stories about your amazing experiences in and on the water. I think you should write a book. What better time to begin than now? Have a great week."

Then, a few weeks later, I wrote, "Hi, Ned, I'm back from Illinois and a splendid visit with my folks. So, what's new in your world? Still interested in a Gulf swim this week? Gosh! A second meeting! This is a first for me. Is this common on this dating site? Or are first dates usually last dates? I'll meet you at the beach. How about if I make a couple deli-turkey sandwiches? Bring your own beverage. Did you do any writing or thinking about that book of yours this past week? Looking forward to seeing you again. Mainly because I never swim alone in the Gulf. You know the old saw. Always swim in the ocean with two things: a friend and a knife. Then, if you see a shark, stab your friend, and swim like hell."

After our beach date, Ned wrote, "Hi, Pat. Thanks for allowing me to join you at the beach today. I had a lot of fun being with you and look forward to our next outing, beach, or lunch. I'll be trying the writing out to see how it goes. You are enjoyable to be with. We have great conversations. Thanks for bringing the sun umbrella. It made the day."

My response said, "Just back from my 11-mile bike ride. One-third of my daily triathlon under my belt. Except I never, ever do the running part so I guess I'm just two-thirds of a real woman."

Ned offered in return, "Congratulations on the bike ride, but I don't buy that two-thirds of a real woman stuff! Seem to be 100% to me! Have a good day, Ned."

Then, I replied, "What I like are the interesting discussions you and I seem to be able to have so easily. You know a lot more about politics, world religions, world travel, the oceans, and life in general than I do, and I can't tell you how refreshing it is for me to have a smart, laid-back someone to talk to. I'm now starting to realize that perhaps I spent the last six years with the same guy mainly because it was convenient being with someone who lived so close. I learned a good lesson."

Then, it was Ned's turn: "I like your intellect and inquiring mind, respecting very much your ability to create and hold a discussion on topics of interest, even those you may not have experienced as fully as I. I'm happy to talk with you and feel no pressure. It's nice to no longer have the stress of direct experience with the nuances of proving one's value. I like you for being at ease with me and letting me experience that ease with my inner feelings. Tuesday sounds great: 11:30 at the restaurant, then the beach will be fun. I'll be ready. Hope you have a great day as I look forward to Tuesday. Take care, Ned."

I opened up in return: "I loved your long letter. You said some very nice things, powerful things, important things, smart things. I guess you're just going to have to put up with my going gaga over the fact that you are a smart, thinking, reading, writing, pondering man. I'm used to conversations about nothing. Boring conversations. But no more. I've vowed that any man I let into my life and my psyche must be a smart, thinking, reading man. My brain is happy just knowing I have a friend like you."

Ned's next communication said, "Pat, you are very kind, and I appreciate it. I did write a lot. Scary. I guess I got on a roll but enjoyed it. I would like to get together this weekend and will get back to you. Take care, Ned."

Those conversations all sounded like Ned and I were on the road to happily ever after, but after another month of dating, mostly just swimming in the Gulf of Mexico, Ned and I parted ways. During those long conversations at the beach I began to notice things about him that were on the fringe. I made a list. Oh, by the way, lists are really good when you're dating. Make lots of lists. Anyway, I decided that life is too short to put up with any of the things I had on the Ned list. He was a nice man, intelligent, and a great conversationalist, but the red flags waved before my eyes like swastikas.

1. Doesn't get along well with his kids.

2. Seems to be drifting, at a crossroads in his life. No real goals or ambitions.

3. Drinks every single day. Sometimes started drinking beer at the beach when we were there at 9 a.m.

4. Overweight and not healthy because of inactivity and too much drinking.

5. Member of a few fringe organizations.

6. Seems to be a conspiracy theorist.

7. Smokes an occasional cigar.

8. Lives with his daughter in her apartment.

9. May not even stay in Florida.

10. Owns nothing.

11. Living on disability.

12. No concrete goals or ambitions.

Patricia Lorenz

12

Mr. Underpants

The following are actual e-mails that I wrote just after the first of the year in 2011 to four close friends.

Dear B, H, L, S:

After meeting six extremely unsuitable men from the Internet dating site since August, finally, a friend has fixed me up with someone she actually knows in person. Of course, I have to give you the scoop. It looks promising. Just yesterday my friend Phyllis who lives in one of those beautiful condo buildings right on the Gulf fixed me up on a blind date with a friend of hers who lives in the same building complex.

The four of us are going out this coming Saturday night for dinner. Will (my blind date) is 69 years old, 6'2" and 280 pounds. He has been married four times and has a loud but very small dog that nearly prevented me from hearing what Will was saying on the phone last night when he called for the first time. (Oh, Lord, spare me! I can't stand yapping dogs!) My friend Phyllis who fixed us up is 84, and she met her fourth husband on Match. Com two years ago. He lives in Greenwich Village, NY, and now they do six months here and six months there. She's deliriously happy. She was the editor of the AAA travel magazine for over 30 years, has been to over 200 countries and on over 200 cruises. But I digress.

Will, my date for Saturday night, is an ex-Army guy who worked as a salesman and is now retired. He seems nice on the phone. Just got over chemo for skin cancer on his chin, has bad hips, doesn't exercise, and sounds like he's 90. Oh, goodness, why is dating so difficult? He insisted on picking me up rather than have me drive to the restaurant to meet the three of them. So, at least he's a gentleman, and if he can afford a 3-bedroom condo right on the shore of the Gulf, he should be able to afford to pay for my dinner which none of the guys I've met on the dating site has ever done on the first meeting. Hence, no second meetings for all but one, the swimmer. Remember him? The guy with all the red flags?

Will has two daughters and two sons and is a reformed alcoholic. He has been sober for 15 years but still goes to weekly AA meetings. Oh, he has quite the schedule: Monday, AA meetings; Tuesday, paperwork; Wednesday, golf; Thursday, plays dominoes and even does domino tournaments—very serious about dominoes. At least, Will doesn't smoke; he quit that years ago. He doesn't sound like my Prince Charming, but I'm willing to meet him.

Somehow I think this is going to be the year I meet lots of different men, take notes on all of them, and use them all as characters in my first-ever work of fiction. Let the dating begin!

Pat

Then, I sent the following e-mail to my close friend Brenda at 2 a.m. the morning of January 9, 2011 after I got home from the date.

Hi Brenda:

I had a great time with Will. First, we had dinner with my friend Phyllis and her husband Harvey, the one she met on Match-com. Will picked me up in his fully loaded Lincoln and even paid for dinner, which was delicious.

Then, he took me dancing at the Marriott and bought me a Brandy Alexander. He's an alcoholic who hasn't had a drink for 15 years but still goes to AA and was very gracious about wanting to buy me a drink. He said it doesn't bother him if people he's with drink. He also doesn't smoke. YEAH! He's very nice, was very complimentary, let me do my fair share of talking, and we seem to enjoy many of the same things. He likes art, theater, shows, and travel. He lives on the Gulf in one of those nice buildings just six miles from my condo.

I'm going over to his place to watch the Packer play-off game later today (after I get some sleep) at 4 p.m. He also offered to take me to the airport when I leave for California next week at that very early hour so you may be off the hook on that trip. I'll see how this friendship with him develops, but I can tell you right now that he is really smitten. At least, that's the impression I got. He's a true gentleman, thoughtful, smart, and, well, I can't wait to see him again.

When he brought me home from the date around 12:30, he called me as he was driving home to tell me something he'd forgotten to tell me, and we ended up talking 45 minutes. Hence, the reason I'm still up at 2 a.m.

He's tall, 6'2" and overweight but doesn't look too bad—white hair and white mustache. Very polite and generous. Kinda cute in a way. Kept talking about things he'd like to do and places he'd like to go with me. Hmm….

Hopefully I'll have lots more about Will to tell you Monday. Please, don't say anything to anyone just yet. I especially do not want Jack to know that I'm dating anyone. OK? Danke.

xoxo

Brenda replied:

Wow, wow, wow! Finally, a date with potential! I am soooooo glad you had such a good time. You deserve someone who can show you a nice time and take care of you a bit. It would be great if this develops further, but take it one day at a time. Don't make faces at the dog! Love the dog! Pet the dog! Befriend the dog! Have fun!

The next morning I wrote to Brenda:

Hey, girlfriend. This is amazing. I woke up this morning at 7 a.m. after five hours of sleep with a smile on my face, just thinking about the possibilities that life has to offer. All the other men I've met through the online personals since August were total duds. I did not go home from any first meeting with any desire to see any of them again. All of them were one-time-only meetings except Ned, the guy I swam in the Gulf with. I went out with him because he was smart, but the red flags kept popping up.

Okay, back to Will. He's smart, lots of common sense, rose up to management in his company but doesn't brag about it. He's got money, or he wouldn't be living for 15 years in that Gulf condo. Not that money matters a whit to me but it's nice to know I wouldn't have to support him. No college education, but he's smart, lots of common sense. We talked politics, world events, and religion. He's knowledgeable but not pushy about it. A decent conversationalist.

Best of all, he likes me for who I am. He's very complimentary but not with smarmy, fake, get-you-into-bed compliments. His compliments are very directed toward me. He loved my painted jars and noticed them right away when he was in my condo for perhaps 90 seconds before we left for dinner last night. He mentioned to Harvey (Phyllis's new husband) late into our 2-hour dinner that the two of them were with two very smart, very talented women. Two different times, he offered me his jacket when we were outside in the cold. He opened the car door when I got in, and when I jumped out on my own when we arrived, I said, "I love it when you open it for me when I'm getting in, but I'd rather just get out on my own. I'm used to that." He understood and was fine with it.

He heard me say on the phone two nights before our date that I don't drink soda and rarely drink booze. Rather, I usually order water with lemon. So, at Marlin Darlin, you know how they have bottles of water on the table? He asked the waiter to bring me a lemon without asking me. He remembered what I'd said on the phone. Imagine that! A man who pays attention! Gosh, this could be something!

All evening he kept asking me what kinds of things I like to do. We have very similar interests. I foresee a very nice friendship with this guy, and it won't be long before Paul, Will, you, and I will be having dinner together at Mango's so you can meet him.

When he took me home last night after dinner we were talking about the play-off game tomorrow night. My beloved Packers are playing with great hopes of ending up in the Super Bowl. I can't wait to see that game. As you know, the Green Bay Packers are the only team I ever watch. Must be those 24 years I lived in Milwaukee. At any rate, the play-off game is tomorrow, and Will asked if I'd like to watch it with him. Heck, yes! So, we made plans to watch it at his place. I offered to bring a pot of chili and a salad that we could eat at half-time. He was thrilled. So, our second date is this afternoon at 4 p.m. Game starts at 4:30, but he suggested I come at 4 so we'd have time for a short walk on the beach in front of his condo. Yes! Should be fun. So, my dear, I'm sorry to say we'll have to cancel our regular Sunday night date to watch *Desperate Housewives*.

About his dog. Last night at 1 a.m. after he dropped me off, Will called me from his car and then again when he got home to tell me he'd checked his odometer and it's only six miles from my condo to his. I said that's a nice distance for a bike ride. We talked for 45 minutes. I like this guy.

When we were on the phone, I didn't hear one peep out of the dog, and he was getting ready to take him for a walk. Clearly, the dog must not yap at 80 decibels all the time so I'll try to be nice. Will already knows I'm not a dog fan and even offered to put Mickey in a different room while we watch the play-off game, but I'm going in with a positive dog attitude, I promise. I'll be nice. This guy is so sweet I wish I could knit. I'd knit the doggone dog a sweater before I go over today to watch the game if I could.

OK, that's it from *Pat's Boring Love Life Central.*

Oh...except that you might find this interesting. Since July when I decided that I didn't want to be alone and that I really do love having a man in my life, I started praying one specific prayer: *Lord, please send me a man who will truly cherish me, someone I will truly cherish as well. And if you can swing it, a man who lives in a beautiful place right on the Gulf of Mexico not too far from my neighborhood would be very nice.* Will is only six miles away. I'm going to bike over there next week one day and see if I like the ride.

I can't wait for you to meet him. I think he looks older than 69, actually, but maybe not. He's kind, considerate and interesting so I don't care what he looks like. He's tall, that's for sure, and after meeting all six of the short online men who were my height, I now realize how much I like a tall man.

I am happy. At noon, I'm taking Norma's son to the airport. Then, at 3:45 I'm driving over to Will's, bringing my leftover chili to eat during the game. I can't wait to see him again.

Suddenly, I can't wipe this smile off my face. As a token of my affection for Will and my Packer fan status, I'm giving him a photo of me today. It's one of my note-card photos in the Packer cheesehead and Billy-Bob teeth & nerd glasses. I hope he loves it.

More from *Pat's-got-a-hot-one* later tonight.

xoxoxo

I arrived at Will's house at exactly 4:05. Four hours and forty-five minutes later, I was on my way home from Will's house. I called Brenda on the phone. "You have to come over immediately. We're watching *Desperate Housewives*! The date was a nightmare. I'll tell you all about it at my place."

Later, after Brenda left, I sent an e-mail to my friend Phyllis who had fixed me with up Will.

Hi, Phyllis,

I'm sharing this for your eyes only. Please do not repeat any of it to Will, but I just had to tell you.

My time tonight at Will's condo (from 4:05p.m. to 8:45p.m.) to watch the Packer game was a disaster—for me, at least. Remember, I am not a dog lover and, in fact, am not comfortable around most dogs. Mickey jumped on me constantly, at least 500 times when I was standing, sitting on the sofa, fixing dinner in the kitchen, during our meal, and when I was on my way to the bathroom. I spent the entire game trying to keep the dog off me with two sofa pillows.

Have you ever been in his condo? If not, picture the left-over knickknacks from four wives, all the stuff they didn't want. His office is bordering on a hoarder's existence. Piles and piles and piles of papers and clutter everywhere. I'm not a neat freak, mind you, but I could never live like that for one nano-second.

The worst thing of all is that even though I was five minutes late he greeted me at the door with shaving cream all over his face and nothing on but dingy, baggy, tighty-whities. He came to the door naked except for his underwear!! It was not a pretty sight, and I was embarrassed out of my mind. Who wouldn't at least grab a towel in that situation?

I can't go back there again. I know Will is smitten with me, but, honestly, I'm not feeling the chemistry. That dog is his life and, it made me so nervous I couldn't wait to get out of there. It is not a well-behaved dog in any sense. It's obvious that no one will ever come between Will and Mickey, and I would never ever consider trying to do that to him since it's obvious how much he loves the pooch. But I just can't deal with the dog and the major clutter in every room. The fact that he came to the door in his underwear on our second date pretty much tells me what he thinks of women in general. I guess at my age I know what I can and cannot deal with.

Again, please do not mention any of this to Will. There's no hope for a relationship or even a friendship with this man after being in his place this evening. So, my friend, keep playing Matchmaker, and keep your eyes and ears open.

Pat

Phyllis responded that same day.

Pat,

I'm horrified! He got comfortable with you and let himself go, it appears. I never saw that side of him, of course. I'm glad you told me the reasons why. I haven't been there since he was married to Joyce and we were invited for stone crabs one evening with another couple. Joyce kept the condo in good condition, at least in the living room. At that time, she had a little dog but it seems to me she kept it in a cage. Harvey remembers it sitting quietly. When she left, she took the dog with her. He only got this dog six months ago. I do remember his cleaning woman saying the dog is loose in the apartment for hours at a time when Will goes out. I don't know how he could have gotten that attached to it so fast, but I can understand that dog not being well trained. Joyce probably did all the training with the first dog.

My cleaning woman did tell me last Friday that someone Will had met recently had moved in with all her furniture. Then, she left so fast she left half her furniture. I never heard anything about that woman other than that because we were in New York for the previous six months. We came back in November, and a woman acquaintance of mine who had worked for me on the magazine called to say she was back selling real estate. At the same time, Will called and said he was lonely, so I asked her if she'd like a date. On December 5, the four of us went to Bon Appetit for dinner. He took her out for a drink after dinner, and, apparently, they had several dinner dates after that. I didn't see them again until New Year's Eve. By then, she had told him they didn't have any chemistry. I don't know what had happened in between. She wrote me this New Year's message:

Hi again:

New Year's Eve was great with really nice people. Yes, let's keep in touch. I will be in the area weekly. Will just wanted too much too fast. I need to get to know a man, especially at this age, before I get involved. Too bad. Oh, well, there is someone for everyone out there. I will be in touch.

I have no idea what happened between December 5 and New Year's Eve, but you can be sure I'll never fix Will up with anyone again. When he was married to Joyce, he seemed to be under control, and I only knew him as a party animal and at board meetings where he was quite vocal but on the same side that I was, protesting the hotel next door.

More than anything else, I'm disappointed that we don't have a foursome to do things with, but that doesn't preclude our seeing you on your own. We have several other women friends whom we see regularly, and Harvey likes everybody I like so we'll just keep doing fun things together minus a man until we find another appealing one. Apparently, you never really know anything about anyone until you date him.

Harvey was very cool toward my little poodle, Nikolas, in the beginning because he doesn't like dogs and is allergic to cats. It became a joke that he was going to throw him down the garbage chute the way Jack Nicholson did in the movie *As Good As It Gets*, but Nikolas was well-behaved and quiet. In time, Harvey grew to love him as much as I did. He was the one who had to take him to the vet to put him to sleep. I just couldn't do it. It upset Harvey so much he threw up in the taxi on the way home. I'm sure if Nikolas had been a yippy little dog, jumping all over him, he would have hated him, too. He would have said, "Will, keep that damn dog off of me, or I'm going home." You were too polite.

I guess a man living alone can get messy. I can't imagine why that last woman left half of her furniture unless she just wanted to get out of there in a hurry.

My abject apologies for submitting you to that horror. I'll certainly know better in the future and never introduce him to anyone again. I think you'd do him a favor if you told him exactly what turned you off so he would change his behavior before he dates anyone again. He should be getting the message after a couple of women told him they had no chemistry. At least, he could keep his clothes on!

Well, my dear, recover from this indignity. When you get back from California and we get back from our cruise in February, we'll do something fun to make up for it.

Phyllis

I replied to Phyllis:

Phyllis,

Thank you so much for understanding this. Believe me there is no need for any apology on your part. You only saw the Will I saw with you at the restaurant. You've never seen what I saw last night, and I hope you never do.

After our date with you guys, I had such hopes for Will, but honestly, after last night there is no hope whatsoever. It's like he put on a great show for me on Saturday night then Sunday was his normal self. He had a whole day to clean the place up but didn't think enough of me to even make a spot on the huge dining room table for our dinner which he knew I was bringing over to eat during the game, which he kept putting off because he wasn't hungry even though I said I was starving. He did say I could go ahead and eat by myself, but I wasn't about to do that. I'd made a lovely salad at home and brought that and home-made chili, and I wanted the two of us to eat together. Finally, during the third quarter of the game he brought in a dish of Hershey's chocolates and ate fourteen of them. After that, I'm sure he wasn't hungry. As soon as the game ended, I jumped up to get the food ready while he took the dog for a walk. I had to stack the files of papers on the dining room table on top of each other to make a little room for our dishes.

Personally, I think women should stop making excuses for men who live alone. I know lots of men who are neat as a pin and very organized and don't keep crap and clutter all over their environment. Will, unfortunately, isn't one of them.

During the game, he kept asking me to move closer to him. I'd say, "I'm fine right here. I can see you and the TV just fine." Then, at least three times he got up out of the blue and said, "You look like you need a kiss." Before I could stop him, he bent down and kissed my non-responsive mouth. It was gross. Of course, by this time with the damn dog jumping all over me constantly, I mean constantly, I had no desire or inclination to be kissed by anyone, especially him. He kept asking if I wanted my feet rubbed. I said, "No thanks, not today."

Your friend explained it perfectly. *"Will just wanted too much too fast, and I need to get to know a man, especially at this age, before I get involved. Too bad."*

There were so many other things that are far removed from my comfort level that I could share, but what's the point?

Please call me when you and Harvey get home from your cruise. When I look back on that dinner Saturday night, I understand that you and Harvey were the reasons I had such a good time. Will and I actually didn't say that much to each other during dinner. You were the fun companions then. So, I'm fine just going with you two, and, of course, we'll always go "Dutch treat" to keep it simple. If you find another great catch, that's fine, I'll give him a one-night-dinner-date chance to check him out, but if you don't find anyone else for me to date, that's fine too. I'm just as happy enjoying some time with you two.

I do know this: Being with the wrong person is infinitely worse than being with no one at all. Anyone who lives like that is not going to change one iota for any woman, and my skin is still crawling after last night's experience.

I left Will's place at 8:45, called my friend Brenda on the way home (she lives across the street from me), and she and I watched *Desperate Housewives & Brothers & Sisters* until 11:00 together, which was actually more fun than my Packer date with Will. Those are my guilty pleasures on TV, at least on Sunday nights, and Brenda and I usually watch together so her husband can watch football at their place. So, at least my night ended on a better note, and it was fun telling Brenda all about Mr. Underpants.

Do me a favor. Call Will and ask for his e-mail address unless you have it. He was going to give it to me yesterday but forgot. I'd like to have it so I can write him and tell him why I don't want to go out again. I'm not good at these things on the phone. I think you're right. I should tell him some of the reasons.

For now, I just wish I could get the image of him out of my mind—his face covered in shaving cream and his body naked except for those dingy baggy white jockey shorts on an overweight body greeting me at the front door. I may need therapy.

Phyllis, you're a doll, and I can't wait to see you and Harvey again. That in itself makes this all worthwhile.

Hugs from your pal,

Pat

From Phyllis the next Monday:

Did I ever tell you about my first Match.com date just before Harvey came into my life? I had gotten a number of photos of men from Denver, Seattle, and Tucson. I wrote Match.com and told them they must be working from the Sarah Palin book of geography. I wanted somebody from the Clearwater, Florida area. So, they sent me a bunch from around here.

One was from a guy who lived in the Japanese Gardens mobile homes. He wanted to meet me quickly because he wanted to invite me to a dinner dance at the Gardens the next weekend if we hit it off. So, I agreed to meet him for coffee at Panera's on that Sunday night. I was a little skeptical because of the mobile home aspect, but when I told my daughter Linda about him, she said, "Be compassionate, Mom. He's probably as nervous as you are and afraid of rejection so be kind, be sensitive."

Off I went, prepared to be compassionate, kind, and sensitive. I pulled up in front of Panera's and parked in the handicapped parking place. He pulled up at the same time into another handicapped parking spot, but he really needed it. He had one short arm and one short leg and what seemed to be a pinhead besides. I was tempted to just get back into the car and drive away, but I remembered what Linda said. So, I put a smile on my face and strode forward to meet him.

He asked, "Are you hungry? We could have supper instead of coffee." I agreed.

For the next two hours, I was my most dazzling. I told all of my funniest stories. They were so funny, I even laughed myself. I was knocking him dead, for sure. I had never been more charming. Linda would have been proud of me.

As we finished dessert, I looked at him brightly, expectantly, waiting for the invitation to the dinner dance. So what if I had to limp a little to match his foxtrot? I was the compassionate, kind, and sensitive Phyllis.

He looked me in the eye and said matter-of-factly, "Phyllis, I don't think we're a good match."

I was dumbfounded. I was a social failure with the world's least attractive man!!! Where did I go from here?

I drove home in a daze. Where had I gone wrong? How could I tell Linda I had failed? That is how I turned into a mean, insensitive, uncompassionate bitch from that point on. That's how I got Harvey.

And from me:

Phyllis,

That is hilarious, your story about the mobile home guy. What are these men thinking? I'm always trying to be sensitive when I meet a guy and very accommodating. I understand that he may be afraid of rejection, but I guess we have to accept the fact that even after 60 years of age 98% of them still think with their sex organs and not with their brains.

The hilarious part is that probably 90% of that 98% are impotent, anyway, by the time they're as old as we are. So, they're stocking up on Viagra and ready to rock and roll. Spare me. I like sex as much as the next person but only with the right man, a man who is willing to let me set the pace. I bet Will bent in to kiss me at least a dozen times Sunday, and on the few times when I didn't duck fast enough, I can tell you this: I did not enjoy any of those kisses or the attempts because they came too soon, too pushy.

Last night, he said, "I think we have really good chemistry, don't you?"

What the big chicken in me answered was, "I guess." What my real brain was saying was, "If being repulsed by your house, clutter, dog, eating habits, and consideration for a pending visitor to your home, is part of my chemistry, then I guess I'm just sizzling with sparks flying out of every orifice." Why couldn't I say what I was thinking?

In my quest for a life of sanity, I have decided three things:

- I won't date a man with an obnoxious, constantly yapping dog.
- I won't date a man who lives in a trailer park. I lived in two mobile homes when I was in college and swore never again. Never, ever, ever, ever again. I may be a snob, but I still want a real foundation under me, especially here in hurricane country.

- I will insist on going to his home on the second date just to see what he's really like.

Yesterday was such an eye opener for me it gives me the willies to think I may not have known any of this had I not been invited to his place to watch the game. I felt safe doing it, knowing you and Harvey were just a few feet away. I should have hightailed it out of there while he was getting dressed right after I arrived. Damn! I'm getting too slow on the get-aways.

Pat

Note from Phyllis:

I can't seem to get the picture of Will in his underwear out of my mind. It will haunt me for days.

I think your three rules are perfect although I wouldn't mind a dog if he were well behaved. Linda has a big, black, pit bull/lab and a malamute, and I must say they make going to her house for Christmas most unpleasant. They take over the living room couches, and you can hardly find a place to sit. If you push them off, they look like they're about to attack so you just wiggle in next to them. They take turns lying at the foot of the stairs so you have to climb over them to go up or come down, and they bark every 20 minutes to go out the back door or come in, so someone has to get up and let them in and out. She's my daughter. So, what can I do? Because the stairs are so precarious, we are about at the point where we won't go there anymore. Too bad because I love her dearly.

Note from me:

Phyllis,

This whole experience has been good for my soul. I learned a lot about myself in the past two days. Plus, my friends over here are enjoying it to the max. So, send me another victim! Please don't give up on matchmaking.

It's 11:20. Bedtime. Tomorrow I'm going to write the letter to Will to explain why I can't see him again. Hopefully, it will help him make some changes in his life before he starts dating another hopeful woman.

Oh, by the way, Will called while I was gone tonight and simply wanted me to call him back at his home number. Tomorrow's e-mail will suffice I think, and if he calls me again, I'll just tell him to read the e-mail.

G'night,

Pat

My e-mailed note to Will or Wonked-Out Willy as I called him after our second date (known officially to my friends as Mr. Underpants):

Hi, Will,

I had a wonderful time Saturday night on our first date. Absolutely wonderful.

You were kind, polite, generous, considerate, and a good conversationalist. Of course, much of my delight was being introduced to you by my dear friend Phyllis. It was so much fun to hear her funny stories about how, at age 80, she met and married her beloved Harvey.

After our double-date dinner with Phyllis and Harvey, I was happy when you wanted to continue our date, just the two of us, at that quaint little bar overlooking the Intracoastal Waterway. I enjoyed the dances, the drink, and our conversation. I was looking forward to our second date the next day, and, in fact, I think it was my idea that we watch the Packer game together.

The anticipation, unfortunately, did not match the reality of the 4 hours and 40 minutes I spent at your condo. Because I think you are basically a good man who has been dealt some tough blows in life, I'm going to be very, very honest with you and tell you why it's not going to work for us. Hopefully you can avoid similar mistakes in the future and find yourself a wonderful woman.

Will, for that second date we agreed that I would arrive at 4:00 p.m., a half-hour before the game started. That would have given us time to take a short walk on the beach (your idea) or for you to show me your condo or to just have a few minutes to talk before the game. I arrived at 4:05.

A man does *not* open a door for a woman completely naked except for his baggy tighty-whity underwear and with shaving cream all over his face, especially for a woman he has only seen once before. You could at least have wiped off the shaving cream, grabbed a bathrobe or a towel, and made a half-hearted attempt to explain why you were running so late. That greeting was enough to put me in a foul mood for the rest of the day. The next time you invite a woman to your place, make sure you are dressed and make sure the dog is in a room with the door shut until you find out if she likes dogs.

The second thing that turned me off completely is the fact that your beautiful condo is a nightmare of clutter, stacked papers, and disorganization— and is poorly decorated (which could be the result of the stuff that four wives left behind). Will, for the next woman, you *must* get your act together and clean up the clutter. I admit it will be a huge job that probably has you depressed by its very size. Try doing one room a week. Get rid of 80% of everything in that condo if possible, including papers, artwork, and furniture. Having too few things is infinitely better than having too many. Think simplicity.

It hurt my feelings that you didn't even care enough about me to clean off the dining room table, especially since you knew I was bringing food for our supper, which was supposed to be at half-time. I had to stack piles of papers on top of piles of papers just to make room for our salads and chili. I had to do that myself while you walked the dog. Knowing how hungry I was since we didn't eat until after the game, you might have helped with the clutter clean-up before you walked Mickey.

Will, for your next female encounter, knock off all the kissing. Not one of your kisses was welcomed by me on Sunday, and yet you kept at it and at it with the determination of a fireman with a giant water hose trying to put out a cigarette in an ashtray. Overkill. A woman needs to really get to know a man before all that smooching starts. Believe me, when the time is right and if I really like the guy and see a tremendous potential in the relationship, I am a great kisser and a passionate woman, but you will never know that because you were too pushy, too fast, too often. We were watching a football game, for heaven's sake! In the future, don't even bring up the idea of a kiss for at least three dates. Let your date be the person who really wants you to kiss her.

Never ask a woman if you can rub her feet on the second date. That is a very personal, sensual thing, often leading to, well, you get my drift. But you don't do that so early in the get-to-know-you stage. You asked me three times if you could rub my feet. When a woman says "no" the first time, she means "no." Don't get me wrong. I absolutely love to have my feet rubbed. Love it. But only by a man I'm in love with. Trust me, I was definitely not falling for you on that second date.

Last, but not least, is the dog. You and I both know the dog is the reason that I will never, ever be able to come back to your condo. Some people are just not dog lovers. I've never had a dog, and I am very uncomfortable around high-pitched barking, yapping, and jumping dogs who never stop that behavior the entire time you're in their presence. You must have noticed the minute I walked into your condo that I was not comfortable with the dog, mainly because he never stopped jumping on me for four hours and 40 minutes. You should have been a gentleman and put the dog in a room with the door shut. Granted, Mickey has the run of your place all day every day, but I spent 95% of my visit with you protecting myself from him jumping on me, pawing me, licking me, and claw-ing me. I was so stressed out from that dog I want-ed to scream and run out of there, but I'm a polite, considerate woman who was trying very hard to understand how a man could be so much more attentive and concerned about a dog than he was with a new woman in his life, a woman he seemed to like a lot.

I'm sure you are a good man, Will. I admire the many changes for the better that you've made in your life, e.g., dealing with your alcoholism by never drinking, giving up smoking, and the like. We are, however, too different in too many ways to ever make this work, so I'm going to save you the cost of another dinner by breaking it off now. I hope you find someone who is more like you.

As for me, I want a man who eats nutritionally, exercises regularly, is totally capable of living by himself in a neat, clutter-free environment, is ac-tive, and enjoys swimming, outdoor adventures, the theater, arts, movies, festivals, and travel. Hopefully, we'll both find what we're looking for.

I share all this with you, Will, not as a put-down but as a way to help you hit a home run next time you meet a decent woman. Take it slower. Don't bring her to your condo until you're ready proudly to show off your beautiful place. Paint the doors on the lanai where the paint is falling off in huge clumps. Put some soap in the soap dispenser in your guest bathroom. Clean off the kitchen coun-ters. Organize your office. Get rid of all the stacks of papers everywhere, especially on the dining room table. Neatness impresses a woman, Will, not you jumping up every half-hour to give her a slobbery kiss. Impress her with how you live, and let her fall for you naturally. After that is when the kissing begins.

I wish you good luck and am very sorry this didn't work for us. Like I said, you are a good man, a fun guy, and a good conversationalist. With a few tweaks to your lifestyle, I'm sure someday you will find a nice woman.

Pat

Followed by a note to my friend:

Phyllis,

Please do me a huge favor. Call Will, and ask him to check his e-mails. Tell him I told you I sent him a long one. He just tried to call me on my land line (twice) and my cell phone. Thank goodness, I bought a new phone last week with caller ID.

I do not want to talk to him until he's read that letter, and then hopefully he won't want to talk to me. I think I said everything that needs to be said in the letter. I'll paste it below. Please read and delete.

Thank you, my friend,

Pat

And then:

Phyllis,

Just heard Will's phone message, and he did read my e-mail. He apologized and wants to start over. Yeah, maybe in six months when he gets his life and his condo in order and takes the dog to obedience school, which we both know is never going to happen.

P

And after that:

To my Four Amigos:

Will, the Pill, just called on my land line twice and my cell phone once. I am out of breath from doing the happy dance over the fact that I bought my first-ever caller ID phone last week and can now see if its friend or foe, feast or famine on the other line. Of course, I didn't answer any of his calls.

Wonked-Out Willy left a message saying he read my letter. Then he apologized profusely and said he would like to start over from scratch. After I recovered from my laughing fit, I thought to myself, *Yeah, buddy, we'll start again after you complete dog obedience school with Mickey, after you pick up and either toss or file each of the 1,345,947 papers strewn all over your condo, and after you clean up the kitchen, stop buying pastries and crap for your obese body, get rid of 80% of the furniture, knick-knacks, artwork and plethora of dog toys in your condo, scrape the doors of your lanai and repaint them, stop the paranoid kissing, fill the soap dispenser in the guest bath, and get a rectal exam because you obviously have your head up your ass!*

Yeah, *then*, I'll start over with him—in other words, when cows really do begin to fly over the moon. Whew! I feel better now. Thanks for letting me vent.

13

Getting to Know Men
Only on the Phone

During those months I was single and looking, I always wanted to talk to men on the phone before agreeing to go out with them. After all, I wasn't about to waste my time meeting someone in person and be forced to sit through an entire lunch if I knew for certain it would never work. So, after e-mails, phone conversations are a must.

Don't be afraid to chat on the telephone a number of times before you actually agree to meet a man in person. In fact, it's probably a good idea to talk to a man five or six times on the phone before you meet in person. Talking without seeing is a good way to separate the men from the frogs. Think about how the TV show *The Voice* works. Great voices are heard by the judges without the singers being seen by those judges. Sometimes, the way a person looks can affect our decision as to whether we want to date them or not, but if we get to know them on the phone and discover what's in their mind and heart before we see how they really look with their warts, bald head, bad comb-overs, or humped shoulders, we might find a prince under that aging body. At our age especially, it's infinitely more important to know what's in a man's head and heart than what his body looks like. Also, keep in mind that the photos men (and women) put on the dating sites are often ones taken ten years ago, photo-shopped, or just head shots. They don't show the real person.

I talked to quite a few men on the phone during those months I piddled around on the online dating service. I never met any of the following men in person. It's a good idea to talk to men in the safely of your own home before meeting them out in public. Just don't get your hopes up. Read on. Here's my list of phone buddies. Note: many of these conversations were one-time-only.

Jim

Age 61 (and 6'1" tall, so he said), Jim was a victim of Agent Orange and just rambled on about stuff that I didn't understand. I didn't have the heart to lead him on so I excused myself after ringing my own doorbell while holding my phone close to the doorbell speaker. "Sorry, Jim, someone's at the door. Gotta run. Nice talking to you."

Charlie

Age 64, Charlie had a BA degree and worked at Lowes hardware store. Within the first ten minutes of a 12-minute conversation, I discovered that he was extremely conservative politically and financially. He was a big golfer, which I'm not. I couldn't find anything we had in common.

William

Age 62, William said he was 5'7" (my height exactly), which means he's really not a hair taller than 5'5". He liked acting, going to school, and being in the Coast Guard reserve. He gave me his e-mail address, which I never used. I think it was the height thing that turned me off. I know…it was probably a shallow excuse.

Shane

Age 64, Shane lived a good hour from me. Although he kept calling, I kept reminding him that I wasn't interested in a long-distance romance. I have to admit that during those calls I thought about my old boyfriend Jack, just down the walkway from me, 57 steps away. Often, I wished could find someone who lived just as close.

David

Age 62, David was a PhD geeky type, who, after retiring from a career as a college professor, made his living writing crossword puzzles for the *New York Times* and the *LA Times*. He played piano and took power walks. We talked off and on for a few weeks, and in my little journal I taped a tiny piece of paper that I'd cut out of a newspaper. I don't know whom the author was describing, but the words fit David to a tee: "He was a sophisticated rhetorician inebriated with the exuberance of his own verbosity. Without question, his message is always the same old self-serving potpourri of pious piffle."

Indeed, my six or eight phone conversations with David were riddled with his verbosity, but the kicker was that he was living with a friend who wanted him to move out. He kept calling me and finally asked if I would ever consider having a roommate in my condo. Move in with me? Sorry. Not now, not ever. Thank God for caller ID!

Phil

Phil was a year younger than me and liked to bicycle and paddleboard. Good start. I'm a huge bicycle fan. He also loved art and traveling. Whammo! This guy might have potential. We were the same religion: Catholic. The kicker that made his acquaintance a one-phone-call friendship was the fact that he doesn't drive. I wondered immediately why—a DUI perhaps? Driving is a must-do in my long list of things I was looking for in a man. Sheesh, how basic can you get?

Scott

Age 62, Scott did not have a photo of himself in his online dating site. That's scary enough, but then when we were talking on the phone, the red flags just kept coming. First of all, his site was named *Fox Cruzn*. Spare me! A fox out cruising at our age? Grow up! This short (5'8"), sassy, Baptist Italian actually started talking about the two of us taking a bubble bath together within ten minutes of our first and only conversation. Click.

Woody

Woody was 68 but only 5'9" (translation: 5'7"). His having been married 34 years and now being a widower was a plus in my eyes. Being with a man who has been happily married certainly trumps a man divorced two or three times. However, during our 10-minute conversation, he mentioned drinking and meeting for drinks a couple times. Having been married to an abusive alcoholic, I find the hair on my neck standing up when booze is a big topic of conversation.

Ted

Age 60, Ted was four years younger than I was at the time. He had a lot going for him. He liked to travel and dance, which I also enjoy. Ted was a golfer, which I am not although the idea of having a golfer as a partner is appealing to me because he'd be gone for hours at a time once or twice a week, giving me a much-needed break, something that is important in any good relationship. Ted was also a pilot. Fabulous! I love to fly. Then came the kicker. He said he wanted to write a book someday about the lies he had to tell to get rich. He said at one point he was worth over 125 million dollars. Then, he lost most of it. Hmm. I'm not into money, but stupidity gets my goat.

George

Standing tall at 6'2", aka Goldstar, born a year after me in 1946, a former cop, a widower with a BA degree, he represented potential. Yes! We only talked a few minutes before he made an excuse to hang up. Sometimes, the men I talked to clearly decided before I did that they didn't want to meet in person. Okay, fair enough.

Frank

A Catholic widower a year older than I who liked traveling, the arts, and exploring, Frank decided when we were still in the typing-online stage that he didn't even want to talk to me on the phone. I e-mailed him my phone number, but he never called.

Kevin

Age 62 and 6'2", Kevin was a recruiter for a hospital. He lived and worked nearly an hour from me. In the first five minutes of our conversation, I heard those four words every woman longs to hear. "Tell me about you."

I talked; he talked. He called again and again. At times, he made weird suggestive comments about what it would be like if we were a couple, which turned me off completely. However, he was smart and clever so we talked for nearly a month, e-mailed, and had quite a few instant messages going in the late night hours. I was intrigued enough to want to meet him, but twice when he said he was coming to my part of town for a work meeting, he never seemed to want to meet in person. Oh, well!

After a while, I grew tired of his goofy conversations, no doubt occurring after he'd had three or four glasses of wine or beer. We never did meet in person even though we probably talked on the phone off and on for at least two months.

Rick

Rick had been a cop for 30 years; then, he served as a federal agent working with the bomb squad, mail theft, and white collar crime. I was intrigued. His wife had died in her 40's. Now he was a semi-retired private investigator. Sometimes, he spoke to senior groups to help keep them from being victimized. We had a couple really nice conversations on the phone, but Rick evidently wasn't interested in me. I was definitely interested in him, but we never met.

Lee

Lee and I e-mailed back and forth for a couple days. His photo on the website was scary. He said he'd had the long, wide beard since 1979 so I knew that wasn't going anywhere. He'd been married three times for a total of 35 years. I guess it was the beard. I just couldn't bring myself to want to meet this guy in person.

Sometimes by the time you get around to the talking stage they, like Irving, a guy I'd exchanged e-mails with, have already met someone else. At least, Irving was upfront about that. So, we never even got to speak on the phone. Life goes on.

14

Getting to Know Men in Person

After the e-mails and then the phone calls, there were the men I agreed to meet in person, but only after I was 100% sure in my mind that they weren't axe murderers or perverts or after my money, of which there isn't much.

Jim

I met quite a few men during those months after Jack and I broke up. One was a 60-year-old gent named Jim. He lived a couple hours from my home so I was amazed when he asked on the phone if we could meet at a local restaurant just a mile from where I live. The date was set for 1:00 p.m. My car was having some work done on it that day so I had to borrow my Dad's car. At 11:00 a.m., two hours early, Jim called, said he was already at the restaurant, and asked if I could come right over? I was in the middle of a project and didn't have Dad's car at my disposal, but like a stupefied love-lost kitten, I said, "Sure, Jim, I'll try to get there in the next half hour."

On the phone a few days earlier, he had told me he was a yacht broker with a master's degree. He had also told me he'd written a screenplay but had no idea how to get it published. He told me that after I'd mentioned to him that I was a writer with 13 published books. My claim was true.

So, anyway, I finished what I was doing in lickity-split speed, called my dad to see if I could have the car, and raced over to the restaurant. I walked in, looked around, and then walked over to the outside section under the canopy overlooking the Intracoastal Waterway. There, in the middle of the place, was a very fat man with his head on the table, snoring.

Oh, Lord, please don't let it be him, I whined. He was the only man in the place sitting alone so I walked up to him and said, "Jim, is that you?" No response. I said it louder, "Jim?" Nothing. Finally, I shook his shoulder. Hard. He finally dragged his obese head off the table and said, "Huh? Oh, hi. Are you Pat?"

Turns out he wasn't a yacht broker and didn't have a master's degree. He was a property manager at the small trailer park where he lived, and he was fat. Very, very fat. Over 350 pounds, I'm sure. To think on the online dating service his code name was MrHandsome. Believe me, he was not. Not in the least.

After boring me for an hour trying to cover up his lies on the Internet, Jim did not even offer to pay for my lunch of soup and crackers. When I finished eating, I said, "It's been nice meeting you, but I have to get this car back to my Dad. Have a nice drive home." I jumped into my car, shaking my head all the way home, saying over and over, "Dating stinks! Dating stinks!"

Miguel

Of Mexican heritage, Miguel was cute, well-built although too short, Catholic, and originally from Brownsville, Texas. When we met at the bench overlooking the Gulf of Mexico not far from my home, he was easy to listen to. It was a very hot day, and the bench was in the direct sun so after an hour of him talking non-stop and me nodding appropriately, he offered to buy me an iced tea at the tiny beach side restaurant behind the bench. At that moment, a cold drink seemed as welcome as a trip to Paris. I started to think Miguel was the kindest human being I'd ever known.

Later, when Miguel and I walked to the parking lot, he proudly showed me his wheels, an oversize, purple pick-up truck, a very, very bright purple pick-up. After those couple hours of him talking about himself and me listening, he hugged me good-by and said he'd be in touch.

Miguel called that night, the next morning, the next afternoon, the next night, the next morning, and on and on and on, at least three times a day for six days. He prattled on about things so mundane that I honestly can't remember a single thing he told me. In all that time, he never once asked me one question about myself. When he told me on the phone that he thought he was falling for me, I pointed out the one-sidedness of our conversations and bluntly told him it wouldn't work for us and to please stop calling. He did. A week later, I stopped having bad dreams about the color purple.

Norm

Norm's code name in the online personals was MrCuddler. He was not cuddly. He was angry, foul-mouthed, and a definite red neck. He was also a retired fireman from Indiana, which surprised me because I have the utmost respect for men and women who serve our country in the fire and police departments.

Norm was short and very stocky. Unfortunately, he didn't have a nice thing to say about anything or anyone. He yammered on in foul language about his ex-wife most of the time we were together at Steak 'n Shake, but he did buy me a very good chocolate brownie shake. When I said good-by in the parking lot, I told him it wouldn't work out because I thought he really hated women. He snarked something unintelligible and jumped into his red convertible. Whee! Free at last!

Ernie

Ernie was my age, 5'9" and an insurance accountant with a BA degree. Trouble is, he worked and lived an hour from me. We talked on the phone a number of times, and it seemed that we had lots in common, including the fact that he had a boat and I love anything connected with the water. Like me, he had children and grandchildren whom he adored. He seemed to be a good man. After each conversation, I was becoming more and more interested in meeting him.

Of course, Ernie replied, "no" when I asked if he smoked. That was always one of my very first questions when I started talking to a man. I can't be with smokers because I get serious lung infections from secondhand smoke, including from electronic cigarettes. To put it mildly, I hate smoking. None of my friends smoke.

After quite a few phone conversations, Ernie and I decided we wanted to meet each other in person on Christmas Eve no less. None of my family could be with me in Florida that year so I was planning to go to the early Christmas Eve services with my folks. Since they were in their late 80's and early 90's, they wanted to go home early. I knew I'd be home alone by 8:00 p.m. Same with Ernie. He had plans with his son on Christmas Day but nothing going on Christmas Eve. So, silly me, I invited him over, which was the first time ever that I had invited a man to my home before I'd had several dates with him, but Ernie seemed so kind and easy going on the phone that I trusted him completely. Luckily, thank goodness, I was a good judge of character.

Ernie arrived on time, sat in the lanai in one recliner while I sat in the other across from him. We talked and talked. It was an easy, fun conversation, filled with great stories and lots of laughs. I served him Christmas cookies and hot chocolate, but after a couple hours, Ernie started squirming in his chair. He finally said he had to go outside for a while. I asked him, "Why?"

He sheepishly replied, "I told you I didn't smoke. I did quit for a while, but I started again. I want to quit, but it's so hard."

I liked Ernie a lot, but I detest smoking. So, I told him I couldn't date someone who a) lied to me about being a smoker and b) was, indeed, still smoking. The bottom line for me is that I would never consider dating a smoker. So, he hugged me, said he hoped I had a nice Christmas, and headed down the steps to his car where he lit up a cancer stick before he even drove away.

Patricia Lorenz

15

Daniel

Daniel was the most pleasant of all the men I met online. His ad declared that he was 5'11", which meant he was really 5'9". Ladies, listen up! Always deduct two inches from a man's bragging height, especially if he's over 50. Sometimes, the poor guys don't even realize they've shrunk two inches. But at our age, who cares? We older women don't wear heels anymore so chances are we're all pretty much the same height.

Daniel and I had a ton in common: education, divorce, kids, grandkids, travel, swimming, exercise, movies, and making money with our investments. We corresponded daily for a week or so by e-mail, then through quite a few phone conversations. I finally agreed to meet him at a local restaurant for a late breakfast. He was waiting outside with a huge grin when he saw me walk up.

Daniel and I went to festivals together and out to dinner alone and with friends. I biked to his condo five miles away to swim in his community pool. We watched movies together at his condo and at mine. When we weren't together, we e-mailed each other every day. I got to know him so well that I even invited him to join my three grand-children from Ohio and me when I took them to an aquar-ium, museum, and planetarium out of town for the day.

Daniel and I had many dates and lots of long talks. Unfortunately for him, many of my talks were about Jack, the man I'd dated for six years and who still lived 57 steps from me. I blathered on and on about Jack and our lives to-gether and how angry I was that he broke up with me over a complete lack of communication. I even teared up when I told him about the woman Jack had been dating for seven months. Daniel became my sounding board as to why we broke up and whether or not it was the right thing to do. One time, I even said something like, "Sometimes, I think I still love Jack if I could just get over being so angry at him!" Daniel would smile and delicately change the subject. The man was a saint for listening to all my angst. I'm sure his sweet compassion made me like him even more. I trusted him and could feel our friendship growing.

I met Daniel on April 1st. Five weeks later, on May 6th (Thank goodness, I kept a journal on all this!), he told me he was falling in love with me. I stammered something like, "I love you, too, my friend, but as a friend for now. My head and my heart are still just too confused to know what to do." He said he understood and would be patient.

The next month Daniel talked me into joining him on a platonic 3-day adventure to a lovely resort in south Florida a few hours from our home where we swam in the Gulf, went for long bike rides and a boat ride, had glorious dinners in a variety of restaurants, played board games, watched movies, and talked our fool heads off.

After being with him 24-7 for three days, I was pretty sure by the time we returned that I would never be able to fall in love with Daniel no matter how hard I tried. He was the kind of guy you wanted for a close friend, but the chemistry just wasn't there. I suppose the Jack thing kept me from giving Daniel half a chance.

Patricia Lorenz

16

57 Steps to Paradise

Six days after my little mini-vacation with Daniel, I had an encounter with Jack in our community pool across the street from our condos. It was the first time in months that we actually spoke to each other. He approached me in the pool after water aerobics and said he'd had a dream about my family and me. He wanted to talk. I agreed to give him 15 minutes at my condo after lunch.

Five hours later after talking non-stop, crying, laughing, and reminiscing, we were back together. That evening, he ended his relationship with his girlfriend of eight months. The next day, I drove to Daniel's condo, called him from my cell phone, and asked him to come down to the parking lot. I explained what had happened with Jack, gave him a hug, thanked him for the two wonderful months we'd had together, and drove back home to the man I knew I'd been in love with since 2004.

Even after eleven months of bitterness, pain, anger, discovery, and new experiences, Jack and I were able to reconnect. Twelve days later, I left with my brother and sister-in-law for a much anticipated 36-day trip to Alaska. Jack and

I missed each other desperately during those days, but it was one of the best trips of my life. Not only was Alaska incredibly beautiful and fun, it was also a terrific opportunity for Jack and me to really think hard about the possibility of truly reuniting and combining our lives once again.

When I returned, Jack met me at the airport, and I fell into his arms. Somehow, those eleven awful months had indeed melted away, and it felt as if we'd never broken up.

Four months later, in November, Jack got down on bended knee at our favorite restaurant on the shore of the Gulf of Mexico just a few miles from where we live. I said, "Yes," and the following June 16, 2012, Jack and I were married.

It was my third marriage. His second. As I write this, we are into our fourth year as husband and wife, and I say with joy that ours is a good marriage. For this, I have to credit the fact that my third and hopefully final husband and I live in two separate condos. When we got back together, I knew there was no way I could ever give up my condo even if we did get married. We're both on the second floor of a two-story condo building, only 57 steps apart. At my age, I knew I needed my own space and my own sense of independence. I was 66 and Jack was 75 at the time of what we lovingly refer to as our "geezer wedding."

We had no attendants, no ushers, no rehearsal, and no rehearsal dinner. Just the two of us walking down the aisle of our church, hand in hand, married by my cousin Jerry, a monsignor in the Catholic church, with more than 100 of our relatives and friends there for moral support.

After the church ceremony, they all joined us at our condo clubhouse for the most fun wedding reception I've ever attended in my life. We had live music, an open bar, and a spread of mid-afternoon finger food that could have fed an army. My kids, their spouses, my grandkids, brother, sister, their spouses, and one niece surprised us with an elaborate flash mob dance to the song, *Get Down Tonight.* It was a magical day.

Our marriage began and continues in two separate condos. We sleep at his condo, where most of my clothes and jewelry live. Then, we go to water aerobics across the street six days a week from 9 to 10 a.m. and then back to his condo where we have coffee (he) and tea (I) while we read the morning paper. Then, we have a late breakfast. He still eats Frosted Flakes. I make my own granola.

Right after breakfast, it's like I have a job. "'Bye, honey, see you later," and I'm off to the outside walkway, past five other units, and to my condo. I treasure those 57 easy steps because it leads me to the place I call home. It's where I work as a writer and where I prepare my speeches for my other career as a professional speaker. It's where I fix a little snack in the mid-afternoon for myself. Jack, after all, has his own refrigerator and cupboards full of snack foods, the kinds of things I don't eat like hot dogs, white bread, and potato chips.

My condo is where I prepare our evening meal. That's because I like my kitchen and my pots, pans, utensils, and dishes better than his. I also like being in control of having at least one meal a day that's nutritious for both of us. My kitchen is a place filled with lovely spices, bottles of sweet red chili sauce, and a great collection of variously flavored olive oils and balsamic vinegars, condiments that my meat-and-potatoes man wouldn't think of putting on a salad or on fresh veggies.

My condo is where I play on my computer after my workday is done. It's where I read books, pay my bills, paint my toenails, organize my stuff, make photo albums, read my mail, create hundreds of paintings with alcohol inks, paint jars, and watch the TV shows that I enjoy. If there isn't a ballgame on TV after dinner, my husband will come into my lanai, where my only TV lives, and watch a show or two with me, but the minute a baseball, football, hockey, or basketball game comes on, he gets that look in his eye. I smile sincerely at my beloved husband and say, "'Bye, honey. See you around 11. Or maybe I'll be over earlier, and we can play cards while you watch the game.'"

I can almost see the relief in his eyes as he gets up from one of the two recliners in my lanai and practically trots out the front door, down those 57 steps to one of his three TV sets where he can settle in and do what God put him on this earth to do: watch sports from a recliner. In fact, at Jack's retirement party years ago, Jane, his beloved wife of 43 years, regaled the audience by telling them that Jack was "a recliner that farts."

Jack and his first wife had a wonderful, happy marriage, and, to be perfectly honest, that is one reason I finally agreed to marry him. He's a good person who knows how to make a marriage happy and calm. When he agreed that we would live in both condos, I knew he was a keeper.

At our ages, another thing I didn't feel like combining was our names. I just couldn't face the work of changing my name again. Like many couples our age who had been married before, I wasn't about to change all my medical, financial, social security, insurance, business, social, church, library, tax, voting, credit card, and passport records. Besides, as the author of 14 books, my byline is pretty important to me, and I'm keeping it forever, thank you.

As I related earlier, when I moved to Florida in 2004, I left a 6-bedroom home in Oak Creek, Wisconsin, the home where had I lived for 24 years and where I raised my four children until they were fully grown, out of college, and on their own. So, I sold or gave away 2/3 of everything I owned. Thank goodness, my children wanted some of my things because now I can visit those treasures in California, Ohio and Wisconsin.

Because of all that purging, when I moved into my condo in Florida, I brought only the things I loved and wanted around me for the rest of my life, including some antiques and heirloom furniture that my parents had given me during my early married life. I wanted to display the hundreds of brightly colored painted jars I'd made over the years. I wanted my crock collection: over a dozen crocks in sizes from one gallon up to 25 gallons. Three of those crocks, the 25-, 20- and 12-gallon crocks, are used as end tables in my living room. My dad made round, solid oak tops for them, and they are not only utilitarian because they store my out-of-season decorations, but they are also great conversation starters.

Jack, on the other hand, is a more modern-furniture kind of guy. He actually has good taste when it comes to decorating. It's just not my taste. So, why shouldn't he be in charge of decorating his condo and I be in charge of mine? It sure works for us.

Another reason we live in two condos is that after raising four children, mostly as a single parent, and spending most of my life running, running, running to various activities those four kids were involved in, and then running a crash pad for all those airline pilots in my home for ten years, I have come to discover that I love being alone. Alone in a quiet condo. No music, no TV, just me and whatever I want to do.

As a woman who can organize a dozen people to meet for lunch or dinner at various restaurants, yuck it up every day at water aerobics class, and speak from the podium to 300 women and chitchat with them later, I find it an enigma that I often cherish the opportunity to be a loner in my own home for a large part of each day. I think every person needs time alone, men and women alike. Perhaps I need alone time because I've been head of my household since 1985 when my second husband moved out. I'm used to making my own decisions and spending my days working in my own environment.

I'm sure Jack would say the same thing about his alone time during the day. As president of our condo association, president of the small pool and clubhouse association and head usher at our church, he has plenty to keep him busy during the day in his own condo…not to mention all those news and sports TV shows he watches.

Don't get me wrong. I love my husband with all my heart and enjoy the time we spend together, always from 11 p.m. until 11 a.m., and often more than that. We're back and forth between the two condos three or four times a day. Jack usually brings my mail over mid-afternoon and stops for a chat in my writing-room office. Or I stop by his place to put on my swimsuit so we can go for an afternoon swim together. Sometimes, we go see a movie mid-afternoon. Or we run errands together. Sometimes, it's as if our two condos are just one big house with a 57-step hallway in between.

The fact remains, though, that I love being head of my household. I like knowing that I can buy new bookshelves for my office or expensive new windows without even discussing the price with Jack. I pay for everything that involves my condo, and he pays for everything in his. When one or both of us has the need to be alone, we can do it without hurting the other's feelings. If I had to watch Jack watch sports on TV so many hours a day I'd scream and think he needed to get a life. This way, we each have our own space that we're in charge of. We can do exactly what we want in our own homes. By late afternoon, I always look forward to seeing my man come in the door to have dinner with me.

I think he's happy, too, to hear me come in his door at night, ready to relax, stretch out on our comfy king-size bed, and do what we have done every night of our married life: kiss goodnight and reach for each other's hand before falling asleep.

Epilogue
Salute to Singles

More than 44% of all adults over 18 in the United States are single: some never married, some divorced, and some widowed. Like many people in this country, I've lived a see-saw life between singlehood and marriage. First, I was single. Then, I was married. Then single. Then married. Then single. Then married. Three single periods in my life. The first time, from birth to marriage, lasted 23 years. The second time I was single lasted a little less than three years. The third single period in my life lasted from 1985 when my second husband and I separated until I remarried in 2012—27 years. I've been single a lot longer in my adult life than I have been married.

If you're single and looking for Mr. Someone Special to fill your life with joy, please remember that coupling and/or marriage isn't for everyone. You can most certainly carve out a life of joy, fun, excitement, adventure, companionship, and fulfillment without being attached to a man.

No matter what you decide, I hope that you will celebrate your life. If you're single, rejoice in it. Too many singles of all ages spend their single lives *in waiting.* They wait for that wonderful day when they'll meet the man or woman of their dreams so they can tie the knot (again) and spend their days in hand-holding bliss. Please, don't spend your life waiting for something better. If you're dating and truly do want to find a partner, spouse or whatever, that's fine. Just don't lose yourself in the meantime. Enjoy your single life status.

Here are a few things you can enjoy when you're single but not necessarily when you're in a committed relationship. You can sleep in the middle of the bed if you want. There's only one alarm clock in your bedroom to irritate you in the wee hours. Toothpaste is always rolled up the way you like. You don't have to pick up after another adult. Your favorite healthy cereal doesn't disappear after two days. You can spend time with your friends and relatives any time you want for as long as you want. You get to make all the decisions without long discussions or arguments. You can purchase anything you want anytime you want. You never have to drive around for hours with someone who refuses to ask for directions. You don't have to feel guilty for being in control of the checkbook. The car seat is always in the right position. You get to be head of household without any arguments. There's nobody at home telling you what to do, how to do it, when it do it, or how much money you can spend doing it. You can cook what you want when you want, including having popcorn for lunch or eating your dessert first. You can cook twice a week and eat leftovers the rest of the time. You can go out to eat every night if you've had it with cooking. You can rearrange the furniture any way you want as often as you want. You can tear whatever you want out of the newspaper even if you're the first person to read it. Your friends can drop into your home anytime without an invitation, and nobody's going to get upset. You never have to wait for your spouse to get out of the bathroom so you can get ready. You can clean house as much or as little as you want. No one will keep reminding you that you've put on a few pounds. You never have to balance your checkbook if you don't want to. No one is going to throw a fit if you put a little dent in the car. You can eat cookies in bed and listen to the radio at 3:00am without bothering anybody.

Here's to the 44% of all the adults in America who are single. May your life journey, whether you choose to look for a partner or not, be happy, healthy, fulfilled and down-right joyful. Life is short. Spend it being you, the authentic amazing you.

-END-

Patricia Lorenz

Appendix A

QUESTIONS TO ASK MEN WHEN YOU'RE DATING

This list of 30 questions to ask a man when you're dating may seem a bit daunting. You're probably saying, "I can't start asking him question after question. It'll scare him away!" Of course it will, but not if you take ten different dates to get all the questions out. Ask three questions per date. Make a photocopy of this list, and cut it up into ten sections with three questions per section. Take the questions with you when you go out for dinner. If you forget the three questions while you're chowing down on shrimp barbie or tofu delight, you can excuse yourself, go to the restroom, and reread your list of three questions. Besides, it's nice to have an emergency conversation starter if you begin to notice uncomfortable silences during dinner.

1. Are you willing to be 100% honest with me?

2. Ever been arrested?

3. Have any pets? Will you travel without them?

4. Ever done or do you use recreational drugs?

5. Are you into pornography?

6. What time do you go to bed and get up in the morning?

7. Are you willing to get off all Internet dating sites completely while we're seeing each other? Or are you still looking for someone else while we're trying to get to know each other?

8. What's the one thing you like about yourself the most?

9. If you could change one thing about yourself, what would it be?

10. What's the first thing you notice in a person of the opposite sex?

11. Any specific personality traits you'd like in your life partner?

12. What do you appreciate most about your life?

13. What are three important things you'd include in your things-you-want-to-do-or-accomplish in your life?

14. Any regrets from your life or past relationships?

15. What do you like to do in your spare time or on weekends?

16. Ever been in a really bad relationship?

17. Do you get along well with your immediate family and other relatives?

18. Why do you think someone would want to get into a relationship with you?

19. Do you like children and having them around you for extended periods of time?

20. Do you ever see yourself getting married again?

21. Why do you think your marriage failed?

22. What is your faith life like? Attend church regularly?

23. Tell me about your best friend. What are your other friends like? How often do you like to get together with them?

24. Do you snore? Suffer from sleep apnea?

25. What kind of foods you like? Do you cook?

26. Do you make your bed every day? Do your own cleaning?

27. How often do you travel for pleasure?

28. Do you think if two people are in a committed relationship that they can each do things separately with friends without the other?

29. Do you belong to any organizations? Business? Pleasure? Church?

30. Since you're retired how do you fill the hours in an ordinary day?

Patricia Lorenz

Appendix B

THE ZERO FACTORS

This is another list you might want to copy and keep with you at all times. This alone is worth the price of the book. I am going to give you 36 good reasons for not starting a relationship with someone. If you're already in a relationship with someone who exhibits quite a few of these characteristics, think about ending it.

Trust me. I'm old enough to know that no matter how old you are, you're never too old for love. The kind of love I'm talking about is dating, romance, living-close-to-each-other love, and caring for each other in a way that transcends small idiosyncrasies, minor fights, and old-age health problems. For some, falling in love at an older age means caring for each other as marriage partners in later years when "in sickness and in health" is often more about sickness. Because it takes so much gumption to forge ahead in a relationship where one person is sick, infirm, or struggling in any way physically, you certainly don't want any major relationship problems clouding the picture and making things even worse.

The more you date, the easier it is to spot the zero factors head on. Once you've had a husband or two, have dated a dozen or more men, and, most of all, have advanced to the ripe and wise age of 60 and beyond, you can usually spot the zero factors like a blinding light coming at you in a train tunnel.

The zero factors are the secrets of dating whether you're 18 or 88. If you're looking for a mate, a significant other, or just a very close friend who has your back, the zero factors are very helpful.

As a woman who did not want to grow old alone but who has a reasonably tough standard when it comes to a potential mate, I had many years of experience meeting men over a cup of tea or lunch in a very public place. How did I know if I want to see the gentleman again? Simple. The Zero Factors, the 37 neon signs that start flashing in your brain at some point in the get-to-know-you stage.

Sometimes, the zero factors pop up within minutes of your meeting. Often, a 2-hour chat in a coffee shop is all you need to see if Mr. Possibility will become Mr. Maybe, Mr. I-Hear-Wedding-Bells or Mr. Quick-Let-Me-Out-Of-Here-So-I-Can-Forget-This-Date-Ever-Happened.

Sometimes, it takes weeks or months to spot some of these zero factors. Many of the examples below came about for me after being with one particular man for a number of years. With that in mind, I just pray that you never, ever jump into marriage with a man you haven't spent a great deal of time with, a man who may start popping zero factors into your face like fireworks months or even years after you start dating.

The Zero Factors work for both men and women. Hopefully, if he has any of these factors in his psyche, you'll be able to spot them in the first e-mails or phone calls before you actually meet in person, but if they pop out into broad daylight on your first date, the list below should help you decide, when he asks for your phone number, whether you want to give him the real thing or the number for Dial-a-Prayer. I'm serious here. I've given a number of men the Dial-a-Prayer phone number. In fact, it's a good idea to keep the number on a small piece of paper in your purse or pocket for that magic moment at the end of the date when he asks for your number. If you never want to see or hear from him again, at least you'll be leaving him with a friendly prayer.

The Zero Factors are kegs of dynamite. If the person you're having coffee or tea with possesses some of these powder kegs, he or she gets a zero. That's it. You're outta there. They are listed below in no particular order.

1. Racist

You can tell right away by the language. Usually, the dead giveaway is an unnatural use of the phrase "white people." Sometimes, they go so far as to use the word "colored" when referring to people of another race. If you hear those words, excuse yourself, and head for the nearest exit.

2. Dishonest

Suppose you've invested two hours with a man who told you he was divorced and you're starting to think that he was meant to be on page one of your book of life. When you ask him how long he's been divorced, he says sheepishly, "Well, I'm in the process. We just separated last week." Bing, bang, boom. Zero! Not only is he dishonest, but he needs six months to a year to get his life back in order and find out who he is before he even thinks about dating and starting over with you or anyone. Of course, dishonesty covers a lot of ground. If you let the relationship get started and even if you learn three months later that he cheats on his income taxes, tells lies about his other relationships, or manifests any other breach of simple honesty, put a big red X next to this zero factor and head for the nearest exit.

3. Shallow

I can't tell you how many men ask women during the first phone call how tall they are, how much they weigh, what they look like, and what dress size they wear. Of course, this is a dead giveaway that he's much more interested in eye candy than having a real relationship with a real woman. Unless you're built like a Barbie Doll, you don't stand a chance with these guys so slam down the zero factor hammer immediately. The funny thing is that at our age he's probably no prize in the looks department, either. Show me a man over 60, and I'll show you bad comb-overs, pot bellies, sagging skin, and slow walkers from aching knees and hips. Looks should not be your or his number one concern because aging takes a lot out of us. We middle-agers and seniors have hearts and minds of gold. We have wisdom out the wazoo, and that's what counts.

4. Mis-yoked

They say your faith life should be similar for a real relationship to work. So, if he's a conservative, born-again Christian fundamentalist and you're a member of a reformed Jewish sect, chances are you aren't going to be happy together at church. If you're into church potluck dinners and choir practice and he's a devout chanting Buddhist, chances are you won't grow together in your faith life.

What you believe spiritually is what you believe. It speaks to the very core of your existence. I'm not sure it's wise to expect one of you to change those deep basic faith roots. My first husband was Methodist. I did marry a Catholic the second time around because I am a cradle Catholic, educated by nuns for 14 years. Our mutual faith was a strong point in our marriage, but, in the end, the 17-year difference in our ages and the fact that we were two totally different personality types no doubt brought an end to that marriage.

My step-mother is Lutheran and my dad Catholic. They take turns. One Sunday they attend the Lutheran church, and the next Sunday they attend Catholic Mass. It's worked for them for over 30 years mainly because Lutherans are basically Catholic-lite. Generally speaking, though, if your faith life is so different there are chasms between your beliefs and his, you've encountered a zero factor.

5. Cheap

I once spent 2 ½ hours in a restaurant with a man who ordered nothing but water. I had hot tea, and the waitress couldn't have been nicer, keeping him filled up with ice water and me with more hot water and an extra tea-bag. When we left, not only did he not even offer to buy my tea, but he didn't even leave a tip for the waitress. I took care of both, making sure she got more for the tip than the cost of the tea, and although I would have expected to pay for my own beverage or food if I'd ordered any, a man always gets rave reviews when he at least offers to pay on the first meeting. Being fair when it comes to dating is one thing; being cheap to the point of trying to squeeze copper out of a penny is another. Speaking of waitresses, I always put a lot of stock in how a man treats them. If he's condescending, argumentative, or demanding in a restaurant, that's a big goose-egg. A man who is kind to every waitress or waiter even if the service is bad is a keeper. It shows that he understands they have a very difficult, tiring, stress-filled job and he's willing to cut them some slack.

6. Homophobic

We have entered the age where being homophobic is as bad as being racist. In today's world, if you believe anything other than the fact that all people are free to love whom they choose and should be free to marry whom they choose, you will stir up a hornet's nest that you cannot win. I believe that since God created all of us, gay and straight, that both persuasions are normal and perfectly acceptable. Unlike some people, I know without a doubt that I was not put on this earth to judge any other human being. When someone does, as in someone you just met on a date, it's time to get out of there.

7. Heavy Drinker

Having been married to an alcoholic, all I can say is please, please, please, please, please, don't go there. The pain is hard to describe. Believe me, the pain an alcoholic causes does not get any better. It only gets worse. Much, much worse. Why even take one step down that path? Unless your alcoholic is a reformed drinker who is still attending AA meetings, has completed his or her Twelve Step program with gusto and grace, and hasn't had a drop to drink for years, do not, repeat, do not date a heavy drinker. Or a drug abuser. Do not. Are you listening?

8. Ex-Basher

Why is it that so many date partners spend their time bashing their ex? Chances are, that ex is the other parent of his or her children. They should be able to get along for the kids' sake. Can you imagine what the basher will be saying about you if things don't work out?

9. Smoker

Smoking is slow-motion suicide, not only for the smoker but also, because of secondhand smoke, for you.

Why on earth would you want to start a new life or a close relationship with someone who thinks so little of himself and so little of you? Smoking stinks. Kissing a smoker is like licking the bottom of a dirty ashtray.

10. No Sense of Humor

If I can't make him laugh or he can't make me at least smile broadly, the relationship doesn't have a chance in the world. Remember, a sense of humor, not only helps solve most of life's problems but is also a boon to your good health. Follow this creed: No laughing, no loving.

11. Hurtful

If he does or says hurtful things, think about whether or not you want to spend the rest of your life with someone who is not kind-hearted. One time a man I was in love with for a number of years actually broke up with me twice when he was driving me to the airport. I was leaving alone to go on special trips, once to California to visit my daughter and once to Hong Kong on an adventure of a lifetime with my brother and sister-in-law. This guy's cowardly way of settling a disagreement (by waiting until I was on my way out of town) was extremely hurtful, especially when I learned the reason for the break-ups months later. Seems he simply wanted to date another woman while I was gone, which he did, but the minute I returned from my trips he asked for forgiveness and wanted me back in his life.

That same man was deathly afraid of conflict or disagreement, called it *nagging*, and after not saying a word, would end our relationship out of the blue weeks or months after I had tried to discuss a problem in our relationship. The point is, behavior like he exhibited on the way to the airport is immature, cowardly, and extremely hurtful. At our age, we don't need hurtful. We need and should expect consideration and joy in our relationships.

12. Thoughtless

At any point in time, any of us can be thoughtless. We just don't think things out before speaking or acting. Once the same man in # 11 broke up with me when I was at a very low point of my life: I had suddenly developed serious vision problems. A real man worth keeping is not someone who will kick you when you're down. So, ladies, beware! If he's thoughtless when things are going okay, you might be amazed what he'll do when the chips are down.

My friend Dianne (born in 1946) told me about an old boyfriend of hers who wanted to start dating her again. Only he wanted it on his terms—mostly he wanted her in his arms just when he happened to be in town. As a former airline pilot, he could travel anywhere he wanted as often as he wanted. She agreed to meet him, listened to his "let's get together every once-in-a-while, including bedroom benefits," spiel. As she thought about his offer, she realized her own self-esteem was at stake here. Then, a small insignificant thing happened when they went out for dinner to discuss the possibility of reuniting. Even though he knew she loved raisin bread, he grabbed the only piece of raisin bread in the bread basket without even thinking to ask if she wanted half. Sure, it's a silly thing, but his thoughtless act was a defining moment for her. The man was thoughtless in more ways than one. Mostly he was thoughtless because all he wanted her for was as a friend with benefits. Definitely not a keeper. It was their last meeting.

13. Sports Nut

Have you ever been with a man who spends most of his free time in front of the TV watching sports? I'm married to one, and one of the ways I survive is by having my own condo 57 steps away so I can stay in my own digs every evening after dinner while my hunka-hunka-burnin' love goes to his condo to watch sports. The year before Jack and I broke up for those 11 months in 2010 and 2011, I decided to test my theory that he really never gave a thought to doing something with me in the evenings. Every evening for six months I waited for him to suggest that we do something together, something we would both enjoy. It never happened. Not one time. I would have loved to go for a walk, visit friends, play a game, take a class together, go for a bike ride, watch the sunset, take in a concert or a play, go out for ice cream, go dancing, or even do Christmas shopping.

I can hear what you're thinking. Why didn't I suggest any or all of those things? I did before the experiment and have done so many times after we got back together. He's always agreeable, but he rarely if ever comes up with the idea to do anything together after supper. During my experiment, I wanted to learn two things: whether or not I was important enough to him to want to spend time with me away from the TV and whether or not he was creative enough to come up with ideas of things we could do together.

In the end, I learned that although Jack does love me, he also loves sports on TV, and I am never, ever going to change that. I also learned that in our marriage I need to be the social organizer and come up with at least 98% of the things we do together. Now that I've accepted those two facts as concrete aspects of his personality, I'm much happier. I get amazing things accomplished in my own condo in the evenings: writing, painting, letter writing, visiting with friends, talking to my kids on the phone, checking up on Facebook, chores, bill paying, etc. It's okay because my husband is happy and at our age the amount of time we're together in any given day is exactly the right amount of time.

14. Unintelligent

Lack of basic intelligence, including poor grammar skills and word mispronunciations, is, for many women, a real downer. Just like we couples should be yoked similarly when it comes to faith and spirituality, a couple should also be yoked similarly when it comes to basic intelligence, education, and perhaps even curiosity about the world. If he barely got out of high school and you have a PhD in physics and are used to the opera and ballet as your favorite leisure activities, chances are you aren't going to get this romance off the ground.

I once dated a man who continually made the same grammatical mistakes over and over. As an English major in college, it really bothered me, not so much for my sake but because I knew that many of the people he was in constant contact with cringed when he repeated the same mistakes. Early in our dating life, I gently explained to him the correct wording, looked sweetly into his eyes in the confines of his living room, and tried to explain that when he said, "He don't know how to do it" instead of the correct "He doesn't know how to do it," many people would perhaps make an unfair judgment about him because of his grammar mistakes. He was offended that I even brought it up and never made the change. The man had hardly ever read a book in his life and showed little interest in learning anything new. At the very least, keep searching until you find a man with as much intelligence and curiosity about learning and exploring the world as you have.

15. A Nutritional Mess

If your date has a horrible, non-nutritive diet and gets little to no exercise and you are a vegan marathon runner, chances are you're never going to make it together. When I met Jack, his favorite food groups were sugar, pastry, fat, and gravy. I learned early on that I could never function or survive if we had just one kitchen because I try very hard to eat healthy foods and snacks. Jack still buys Frosted Flakes and other sugar-coated cereals, cookies, potato chips, fried foods, gravies, and white bread. We eat breakfast together at his condo every morning, but I have my own foods there: homemade granola, whole grain breads, berries, yogurt, etc. We both love eggs so it's a fun morning when we can enjoy a nice omelette together.

Exercise? My man had never exercised in his life other than the occasional game of golf. However, he always rides a golf cart so that doesn't count much. When we started dating in 2004, I asked him to join me in water aerobics because he loves to be in the pool. He agreed, and today we both still go every morning six days a week for an hour doing vigorous exercises to different aerobic tapes. So, you can teach an old dog new tricks. You just have to be persistent.

Here's something to think about. If you're going to live with or marry a man in your later years, think twice about it if he has many ingrained bad eating habits. Do you want him to take you down the road to poor health and nutrition? Think about how important your health is to you. Try to find someone who has a healthy diet and similar exercise interests.

16. Obese

Believe me, I'm no Barbie Doll. I've gained and lost the same 20 or 30 pounds over and over my entire life. But I try hard to eat healthy foods, and I exercise. Swimming, water aerobics, biking, and walking. If you're dating a man who is obese and most of those 50-100 extra pounds are around his middle, you can plan on being a widow at the end of your life. Look at him when he's standing sideways.

Even 30 extra pounds on a man's middle is not attractive, healthy, or a turn-on in any way.

Sometimes you just have to tell them what you're thinking in terms of their health. When my dad met my future step-mother she was a smoker. When he realized they were falling in love, he told her that he couldn't marry a woman who didn't respect herself enough to not smoke. He didn't ask her to stop smoking for him. He simply made that statement, putting the onus on her. She quit cold turkey and never looked back. They've been happily married since 1982 and are now in their 90's.

17. Shallow Family

It's a simple fact. When you're with a man, you're with his entire family. They become your family. How do you get along? Do they treat you with respect? Do you have interesting, lively discussions with lots of laughs and good times, or do you sit around watching them drink, smoke, argue, and talk about each other? Think about whether or not you'd like to be on a family vacation with these people—his children, grandchildren, brothers, sisters, nieces, and nephews. If the answer is *no, you do not want to consider his relatives as your beloved relatives*, well, then, perhaps this is not a marriage or a relationship you want to consider.

18. Financially Irresponsible

Is he a big spender who spends money on a whim and has little monetary sense when it comes to saving money? At our age that can be a make-it-or-break-it problem. If he's been paying only the interest on his home loan for years or making the bare minimum payments monthly on his credit cards, turn around and run as fast as you can. This is not a man you want to mingle your money with. Sometimes, I think not wanting to mingle money is one of the main reasons so many middle-aged and elderly people do not want to get married in their later years.

There is an alternative to this problem, however. If you do get married in your later years, don't mingle your money. You can have one joint checking account into which you each funnel money every month to pay your common household bills. Otherwise, you pay for your personal items, car expenses, travel, medical bills, and he pays for his. That way neither of you has to worry about how your life savings are going to be spent. Late-in-life marriages tend to work better that way.

So, if he spends money in a totally different way than you do, keep it all separate. If he's living on social security and you've saved your whole life for a nice retirement, don't risk having it disappear in a year or two if he ends up in a nursing home in ten years. See an elder law attorney to draw up papers that will allow him to keep what's his and you to keep what is yours should the unthinkable occur. If continuing in the relationship means it's going to bankrupt you sooner rather than later, rethink the whole marriage thing. Perhaps living together as partners/companions is a better option than getting married.

19. Adventureless

Where in the world has he been? Where would he like to go? Does he have a sense of adventure when it comes to travel, or is he content to go on two or three cruises a year to the same Caribbean Islands? Of course, if that is your idea of fun times, then you're perfect for each other. My Jack loves to cruise and has been to the Caribbean probably 30 times in his life, including 20 times with his first wife. After we got married, I told him I would never go on another cruise to the Caribbean unless he paid for my share. During the first year of our marriage, we drove through five national parks out west after flying to Arizona. The next year, we flew to Ireland and spent three full weeks driving the entire perimeter. The third year, we took a 3-week cruise across the Atlantic, then visited a dozen interesting places including the Azores, Spain, Italy, Sicily and Monaco. It was the most magnificent, interesting, educational cruise of my life, and even Jack is now convinced how much better it is when you can actually do something besides look at tacky gift shops and visit the beach.

If your idea of travel differs greatly from his, at least try it his way and then your way so you can both experience the other's preferences. Then, decide if you're willing to find ways to compromise before you make it a permanent relationship.

20. Stress Phobia

To be with some men means you must walk on eggshells all the time for fear something you say might cause them stress. I once knew a man who was terrified of being stressed about anything so he stuffed his feelings and expected his woman to stuff hers. That's why they sell a lot of antacids, folks. Stuffers—for people who don't know how to talk about their feelings or refuse to for fear it will end in a disagreement. A good discussion with no yelling is the very basis for what a real relationship is all about. A man who is afraid to fight for what he believes is right or is afraid to even talk about what is bothering him is not a real man. The same goes for a woman. If you're afraid to open up, then you're not real.

Talk. Share. Be honest. Discuss. Learn from each other. To avoid stress at all costs? It's crazy. Idiotic. What you're creating is an eggshell instead of a relationship. Take a class in how to fight fairly and with respect for each other. Stress is part of life. Learn to deal with it. If he avoids stress at all costs, excuse yourself, and go find someone you can really get down to the nitty-gritty with.

21. Mean

When a man does not care about your state of mind, health, well-being, or needs and, in fact, does specific things that demonstrate a streak of meanness, you need to get as far away from him as possible. Does he put you down or belittle you to his friends? Does he make you feel used or more like his caretaker than a real relationship partner? Does he criticize your weight, clothes, or hair? Sometimes, it's hard to spot mean because often a man can be on his best behavior until you move in with him, or, heaven forbid, actually tie the knot. Hopefully, mean streaks will appear way before you get that serious. If they do, run like hell.

22. Inability to Connect

A couple must connect on three aspects in a relationship: intellectual, psychological, and physical. Like a tripod, the relationship will eventually fail if one of the legs is weak. Did you ever know a man or woman who was just in the relationship for the physical pleasures it could provide? By physical, I mean a lot more than sex. Some women and/or men stay in relationships because they get to be pampered with more meals in fancy restaurants. Or they like to be driven around in a nice car. Or one of the partners has a nicer home or condo than the other, and it's fun to hang out in the more luxurious place. All bad reasons for staying together. Don't let physical pleasures cover up your inability to connect on an intellectual or psychological level. Come on, what are you going to talk about during those long, luxurious dinners in that fancy restaurant? What happens when your feelings are hurt and you don't have a clue how to open up to him about what's bugging you? If you can't connect in all three ways, it doesn't make sense to try to connect at all. Disconnect.

23. Porn User

I dated a man once whose interest in pornography disgusted me. Quite by accident, two of my relatives discovered hundreds of porn sites that he had visited on his computer. Porn makes a woman feel like an unattractive sexual failure, but what it does to the man himself is even more insidious.

Years ago, I taught a high school religious education class, and we discussed porn in that class because it's so available and so out there for kids today. The one thing that stuck with me is that porn is a progressive deterioration of the porn user's mind, emotions, and relationships. Progressive. That means it doesn't stay the same; it gets worse.

Numerous studies have been done about how pornography is progressive. In other words, users progress to more types of porn, eventually using it for personal sexual fulfillment. The user seeks out more pornographic material, including hard core films, magazines, and eventually moves on to sexual stimulation in strip clubs and adult movie theaters. Next comes sex with prostitutes and/or casual sexual encounters that mean nothing to the man emotionally. For some, the progressive deterioration includes sexual torture, rape, or murder as in the case of famous pornographer and serial killer Ted Bundy. Progressive. It doesn't end with photos in a girly magazine. It progresses insidiously over time until relationships are destroyed completely. Remember, porn is a zero factor.

24. Negativity

Does the man you're contemplating have a negative personality? He sees the glass half empty, notices all the rain clouds in life, and never gets excited or even remotely happy about any new experiences? He grumbles about everything and points out all the negatives. Life is too short to be yoked to a downer.

Physical complaints are another thing to watch out for. Is he constantly complaining about back pain, leg pain, hip pain, shoulder pain, neck, arm, head, or heel pain? Face it. Older folks in their 50s, 60s, 70s, 80s, and beyond certainly do have aches and pains. That's life. There's nothing wrong with giving each other a little sympathy every now and then, but if your intended lover boy is constantly complaining about something or other, back away, and try to find yourself an optimist. Don't let him drag you down a bleak, unhappy road filled with complaints. For sure, his negativity will wear off on you, and you may start to be a complainer about everything as well. Find yourself a happy guy who likes himself and the world and puts a positive spin on things.

25. Not Invested in the Relationship

Does he really need or cherish the relationship you're trying to create? Does he seem aloof about it? If, after every little disagreement or spat, he makes comments like "Find somebody else; be my guest," that most definitely indicates that he isn't truly invested in you for the long haul.

26. No Creativity

Does he have a creative hobby? Can he make anything from scratch, from woodworking to decorative cakes? At the very least, does the man you're considering have plenty of fun, creative ideas of interesting things to do? Or is he just willing to go along with whatever you suggest? If he's content to just sit and watch TV day after day and is not intellectually curious or stimulated about anything in life, you might move on and find someone who does have a creative mind. It's true that women are generally the social organizers for a couple, but you certainly don't want to have to do it 100% of the time. His interests should make your life sizzle as well. Ask him to plan a weekend adventure for the two of you. Then, let him do it. If he just can't figure it out or plan something good for both of you, then perhaps you need to cut him loose.

27 Unaffectionate

If you've been together for a number of dates and he hasn't even tried to kiss you or hold your hand, you may have a deadly dud on your hands. If he's a great kisser and very affectionate but only initiates it in bed with ulterior motives, you two need to have a talk. Foreplay does not begin in the bed. It starts the day or many days before with lots of sweet gestures, hand holding, back rubbing, and a pat on the shoulder. Foreplay is affection without sex in mind as the ultimate goal.

If he never initiates affection for any reason other than intimacy, tell him to get a blow-up doll instead. At our age, we want a man who is affectionate and a great cuddler. Believe me, most men after 50 aren't that good in bed, anyway, unless they're regular visitors to the pharmacy for the little blue pill. Affection goes a long, long way in a relationship, especially if sex is a difficult thing to accomplish for either of you. So, in other words, if he isn't interested in cuddling and touching you, you might need to reconsider this relationship.

28. Bull-headed

If he's really bull-headed and instead of getting into a calm discussion about something he clams up and does it exactly his way every time, it's time to turn him in for a sweet guy who sees it your way some of the time. Compromise is a great virtue.

29. Too Old

If the difference in your ages seems to grow wider the older you both get, find someone closer to your own age. If he's 73 going on 80 and you're 64 going on 50, it probably isn't going to work. A 30-year difference in mental, physical, and emotional ages is way too much. Many women do well with a man a few years her junior once she hits midlife. Just look for someone who is your equal when it comes to the kinds of activities you like to do. If you love to hike, snorkel, and kayak and his idea of sports is watching baseball on TV and the thought of a good hike gives him the heebie jeebies, then you're not on the same page physically. If you can still run, run. Run away, and find someone who enjoys the same kinds of things you do and is physically fit enough to be able to do them.

30. Unwilling to Share Power

Chances are, if you're looking for a good man you've been alone for some time, which means you're head of your household. If you're used to making all the decisions about your home, finances, purchases, repairs, improvements, and the like, it's going to be difficult to co-exist with a man who wants to make all those decisions. Even after you marry or move in together, you still have the right to continue making your own decisions about your home and your life. If he's a chauvinist who thinks the man has all the power, quick, turn around, get out of there, and find a guy who's willing to share.

31. Too Demanding of Your Time

I need to have my own space, home and office where I can be alone a great deal of the time to think, plan and write books. I like being alone. But I'm also a very social person who loves friends and interesting activities when I'm finished writing. Sometimes, I want to do things with my women friends. If the man you're with thinks you should be together 24-7 and even gets jealous of the time you spend with others when he's not included, you may have a big problem on your hands.

32. Few Interests in Common

It's perfectly fine for both of you to have interests that the other could do without for the rest of his or her life. For instance, Jack golfs. I hate golf and will never take up the game, but he enjoys it once a week with his twin brother. I'm grateful that these two brothers get together every week for a wholesome activity that they both enjoy. I like to paint, write, and sometimes travel by myself to visit my children and grandchildren. Jack doesn't begrudge me the time I spend away from him. Truth be told, I'm sure he enjoys his time alone as well so he can do and eat as he wants.

33. The "Mrs." Conflict

If you have plans to keep your name even after you get married, discuss it now while you're dating. In my 60s when I married Jack, I had no intention of ever changing my last name again, and, luckily, Jack understood. It's too much work to make all those dozens of name changes including medical, work, business, church, banks, credit cards, insurance, byline, voting, etc. Many women keep their last names when they marry these days. If he's so old-fashioned that he can't comprehend having a wife who does not also have his name and you desperately want to keep the name you've had most of your life, think twice. If your name defines who you are, don't give up on you. The name change conflict may be a zero factor.

34. Is His Family Unaccepting?

I could never, ever replace Jane as a mother to Jack's kids or grandmother to his grandchildren, and for years it was hard for them to accept me as someone important in their dad's life or their lives. I've been respectful of their feelings and even told Jack that it would never bother me if he talked about his beloved wife Jane in front of me. In fact, we've had many wonderful conversations about his life with her. After all, they were happily married for 43 years before she died. A man who can accomplish that is a keeper in my mind. My relationship with his children got better slowly after we got married. At least, we all get along, have a mutual respect for each other, and do have fun when we're together. However, word of warning: if your man's kids, siblings and grandkids have demonstrated that you will never be accepted in their life, reconsider the relationship. It's very true that when you marry the man, you marry his family. Do you want to be married to his family? If not, get out now while you can.

36. BRAGGERT

Is he always bragging about his past accomplishments, career, lifestyle, wealth, and possessions? Do most of his sentences start with "I"? Does he leave you in the dust when you're needing a little ego boost? Chances are if he's behaving this way when you're dating, you'll just end up listening to the same old bragging stories again and again if you solidify the commitment.

37. Willingness to Settle

If you treasure your independence, don't settle for a committed relationship just because it seems to make your life easier, more comfortable, safer, or less lonely. Settling for a man who is not a good match for you will make you feel like less of a woman soon after the commitment is made. You deserve the man of your dreams, and he's out there. Don't be in such a hurry to shut the book on meeting, greeting, dating, and falling in love slowly.

Final thought: If you are already in a relationship and you're guilty of letting a dead-end relationship linger long past its shelf-life because the task of ending it seems just too difficult and painful, grab yourself by the shoulders and shake them hard. Break up, and get on with your life. You may suffer for a month, six months, or even a year, depending on how close you live to each other. The more you run into each other, the more difficult it is to get over, but a year is better than ten or 20 years of unhappiness or a marriage of mediocrity.

Appendix C

THE PLUS FACTORS

Here, just for your convenience, is a list of the plus factors. In many ways, they are the flip slide of the zero factors.

Make a copy of this list, and keep it handy when you're out there dating. One thing's for certain: you are worth it. Respect yourself enough to keep looking for the man who exhibits all or at least most of these factors. Otherwise, you're better off living alone and having fun with your family, women friends, married couple friends, church friends, neighbors, and work friends. There are many people in your life and it's up to you to get things started with them when you're feeling lonely.

If finding a man is your main goal, a man you can walk into the sunset with, please be careful. Don't rush. Jack was a part of my life for eight years before we got married. Quite frankly, it took me that long to decide that he was the man for me. There's no hurry. Just live your life, be the happiest, kindest person you can possibly be, and if Mr. Wonderful comes across your path, take it easy.

I pray your love will be laced with all or most of these plus factors. Here's the list in no particular order. Keep it handy. Be happy!

Mr. Wonderful has or displays the following traits:

1. Acceptance of all people: race, religion, sexual persuasion, politics

2. Deep thoughts, ideas, dreams

3. Honesty

4. Similarity of or same faith level and/or church affiliation

5. Generosity

6. Social drinking only or is a non-drinker

7. Respect for ex-wife or ex-girlfriends

8. No smoking addiction (i.e. is a non-smoker)

9. Great sense of humor

10. Kindness

11. Thoughtfulness

12. Energetic passion about many things

13. Smartness

14. Nutritious diet

15. Normal body weight or close to it

16. Loving, accepting family members

17. Financial integrity

18. Sense of adventure

19. Ability to handle stress

20. Ability to connect intellectually, psychologically, and physically

21. Lack of interest in porn

22. Positive outlook
23. Commitment to making the relationship work and grow
24. Creativity
25 Affection
26. Willingness to give in on some issues
27. An age the same as or approximate to yours
28. Willingness to share power
29 Non-demanding nature
30. Many interests
31. Similar travel interests and needs
32. Willingness to let you maintain your own identity
33. Acceptance of you by his family
34. Similar ways of spending and saving money as you
35. Humility
36 Unwillingness to settle just to have a warm body nearby
37. Trustworthiness
38. Patience

Other Books by Patricia Lorenz

Positive Quotes for Every Day Publications International Ltd. 2010

Serial Killer's Soul Title Town Publishing 2010

The Five Things We Need To Be Happy Guideposts Books 2009

Daily Devotions for Writers Infinity Publishing 2008

Chicken Soup for the Chocolate Lover's Soul HCI 2007

Chicken Soup for the Tea Lover's Soul HCI 2007

Chicken Soup for the Dieter's Soul Daily Inspirations HCI 2007

True Pilot Stories Infinity Publishing 2005

Life's Too Short to Fold Your Underwear Guideposts Books 2004

Grab the Extinguisher, My Birthday Cake's On Fire! Guideposts Books 2004

Great American Outhouse Stories Infinity Publishing 2004

A Hug a Day for Single Parents Servant Publications 1997

Stuff That Matters for Single Parents Servant Publications 1996

Select MSI Books

SELF-HELP BOOKS

A Woman's Guide to Self-Nurturing (Romer)

Creative Aging: A Baby Boomer's Guide to Successful Living (Vassiliadis & Romer)

Divorced! Survival Techniques for Singles over Forty (Romer)

How to Live from Your Heart (Hucknall)

Living Well with Chronic Illness (Charnas)

Publishing for Smarties: Finding a Publisher (Ham)

Survival of the Caregiver (Snyder)

The Rose and the Sword: How to Balance Your Feminine and Masculine Energies (Bach & Hucknall)

The Widower's Guide to a New Life (Romer)

Widow: A Survival Guide for the First Year (Romer)

INSPIRATIONAL AND RELIGIOUS BOOKS

A Believer-Waiting's First Encounters with God (Mahlou)

A Guide to Bliss: Transforming Your Life through Mind Expansion (Tubali)

El Poder de lo Transpersonal (Ustman)

Everybody's Little Book of Everyday Prayers (MacGregor)

How to Get Happy and Stay That Way: Practical Techniques for Putting Joy into Your Life (Romer)

Joshuanism (Tosto)

Living in Blue Sky Mind: Basic Buddhist Teachings for a Happy Life (Diedrichs)

Puertas a la Eternidad (Ustman)

Surviving Cancer, Healing People: One Cat's Story (Sula)

The Gospel of Damascus (O. Imady)

The Seven Wisdoms of Life: A Journey into the Chakras (Tubali)

*When You're Shoved from the Right, Look to Your Left: Metaphors of
    Islamic Humanism (O. Imady)*

MEMOIRS

Blest Atheist (Mahlou)

Forget the Goal, the Journey Counts . . . 71 Jobs Later (Stites)

Good Blood, 2 volumes (Schaffer)

*Healing from Incest: Intimate Conversations with My Therapist (Hen-
    derson & Emerton)*

It Only Hurts When I Can't Run: One Girl's Story (Parker)

Las Historias de Mi Vida (Ustman)

Losing My Voice and Finding Another (C. Thompson)

Of God, Rattlesnakes, and Okra (Easterling)

Road to Damascus (E. Imady)

FOREIGN CULTURE

Syrian Folktales (M. Imady)

The Rise and Fall of Muslim Civil Society (O. Imady)

*The Subversive Utopia: Louis Kahn and the Question of National Jew-
    ish Style in Jerusalem (Sakr)*

Thoughts without a Title (Henderson)

PSYCHOLOGY & PHILOSOPHY

Anxiety Anonymous: The Big Book on Anxiety Addiction (Ortman)

Depression Anonymous: The Big Book on Depression Addiction
    (Ortman)

Road Map to Power (Husain & Husain)

*The Marriage Whisperer: How to Improve Your Relationship Overnight
    (Pickett)*

HUMOR

PARENTING